Critical Pathway Implementation Guide: A Methodology for Managing Critical Pathways

Deborah K. Wall RN, BSN, MA
Mitchell M. Proyect BA, SD

Precept Press, Chicago
Division of Bonus Books, Inc.

Wall, Deborah K.
Critical pathway implementation guide: a methodology for managing critical pathways/Deborah K. Wall, Mitchell M. Proyect.
p. cm.
Includes bibliographical references and index.
ISBN 0-944496-54-7 (alk. paper)
1. Health services administration. 2. Critical path analysis. 3. Medical care—Quality control. 4. Medical care—Cost control.
I. Proyect, Mitchell M.
RA971.W34 1997
362.1 ' 068—dc21 97-23771
CIP

Precept Press
Division of Bonus Books. Inc.
160 East Illinois Street
Chicago, Illinois 60611

Table of Contents

CHAPTER 1 Reengineering Quality/Resource Activities 1

Introduction 1
Reengineering 1
Reengineering Principles 3
- Focus on Redesigning Processes 4
- Reengineer from the Top Down 5
- Combine Several Tasks into One Job 6
- Perform Work When it Makes the Most Sense 8
- Work Where it Makes the Most Sense 9
- Processes Have Multiple Versions 10

Role of Information Technology in Reengineering 11
Case for Action 12
Vision Statement 14
Reengineering Process 14

CHAPTER 2 Implementation of Critical Pathways 17

Introduction 17
Manage Pathway Implementation 17
- Pathway Implementation Strategies 20
- Lack of Clinician Acceptance 21
- Inconsistent Application of Pathways 21
- Inability to Manage Pathway Data 21

Development of Support Mechanisms 23
- Guidelines or Procedures 23
- Staff Responsibilities 23
- Key Pathway Definitions 24
- Pathway Procedures 25
- Documentation and Recording Systems 26
- Pathway Reference Guides 29
- Pathway Documentation Forms 32
- Patient Education Materials 39

Product and Service Delivery System 41
Provision of Staff Education 42
Orientation to Critical Pathways 42
Skill Building Education 43
Just-in-Time Education 44
Implementation Exercise 45
CHAPTER 3 Measurement of Results 47
Introduction 47
Collection of Pathway Information 47
Assignment of Responsibilities 47
Identification of Pathway Data 49
Measuring Individual Pathway Elements 50
Measuring Reasons for Variance 50
Developing a Variance Identification System 52
Measuring Patient Outcomes 57
Plan Data Collection 57
Timing of Data Collection 57
Data Collection Process 58
Manage Individual Cases 58
Analysis Of Data 59
Pathway Elements 65
Clinicians' Performance 67
Reasons for Variance 67
Patient Outcomes 68
CHAPTER 4 Utilization of Critical Pathway Results 73
Introduction 73
Reinforcement of Desired Performance 73
Positive Reinforcement 74
Results through Feedback 74
Removal of Impediments 75
Identification of Triggers 76
Practitioner Triggers 76
Institutional Triggers 76
Community Triggers 77
Implementing Pathway Revisions 77

Who Can Initiate a Revision? 77
How to Start Pathway Revisions? 79
What Actions Revise a Pathway? 80

CHAPTER 5 Determining Fiscal Impact of Improved Clinical Processes 83
Introduction 83
Determining Financial Health 83
Proving the Cost Benefit of Quality Initiatives 85

CHAPTER 6 Relationship between Critical Pathways and Case Management 91
Introduction 91
Current Case Management Models 92
Relationship between Case Management and Critical Pathways 94

APPENDIX A Pathway Policy and Procedure 97
APPENDIX B Glossary of Terms 105
APPENDIX C Bibliography and References 109

1

Reengineering Quality/ Resource Activities

Introduction

With recent changes in reimbursement strategies, available technology and the Joint Commission's accreditation standards, there is increasing impetus to embrace critical pathways as a tool for controlling clinical costs and promoting quality patient care. But many organizations are finding that pathways can not be created, measured or maintained without reengineering current patient care review activities.

Frequently, the current performance improvement, utilization review, discharge planning and risk management programs are fragmented, causing duplication of data collection, minimal data analysis and the inability to meet the increasing needs for timely data analysis without increasing staff. Many administrators are asking how can this situation be changed?

This chapter was designed to answer this question and to explain how pathways can serve as the cornerstone for reengineering current patient care review activities into an integrated clinical data management process.

Reengineering

One of the new buzz words being used by health care executives and others is the term **reengineering**. Reengineering is "the fundamental rethinking and radical redesign of processes to achieve dramatic improvements in critical, contemporary measures of performance, such as cost, quality, service and speed." Secondly, reengineering is not synonymous with downsizing, automation, restructuring, delayering or total quality management. **Reengineering focuses on what must be**

done and then how to do it. This change is brought about through radical redesign of essential processes which result in dramatic improvements.

Reengineering differs from total quality management in several ways. While quality programs work within the current framework of the organization to make incremental improvements to existing processes, reengineering seeks to reinvent the organization and replace processes. The goal of total quality improvement is to do current processes better. **The goal of reengineering is to invent new approaches to essential health care processes.**

Although reengineering differs from total quality management, there are several similarities. Both processes recognize the importance of process and work backwards from the needs of the process customers.

To start the reengineering of current patient care review processes, we need to determine the intent of each review function. For example, the goal of utilization review is to obtain maximum insurance payments and minimize clinical costs. The goal of quality improvement is to improve patient outcomes and meet the Joint Commission's and other accreditation standards. The goal of risk management is to limit litigations and prevent injuries. The goal of discharge planning is to move patients to alternate levels of care.

The goals of developing and implementing critical pathways is to control clinical costs, maximize reimbursement, improve patient outcomes, limit litigations and move patients rapidly to alternative levels of care. A side benefit of critical pathways is meeting the new integrated performance improvement standards of the Joint Commission and NCQA.

By identifying the common goals for both the current patient care review activities and the critical pathway process, we can start to recognize how pathways can replace many of the current quality and utilization activities without failing to meet customer needs.

What Needs to Be Accomplished?

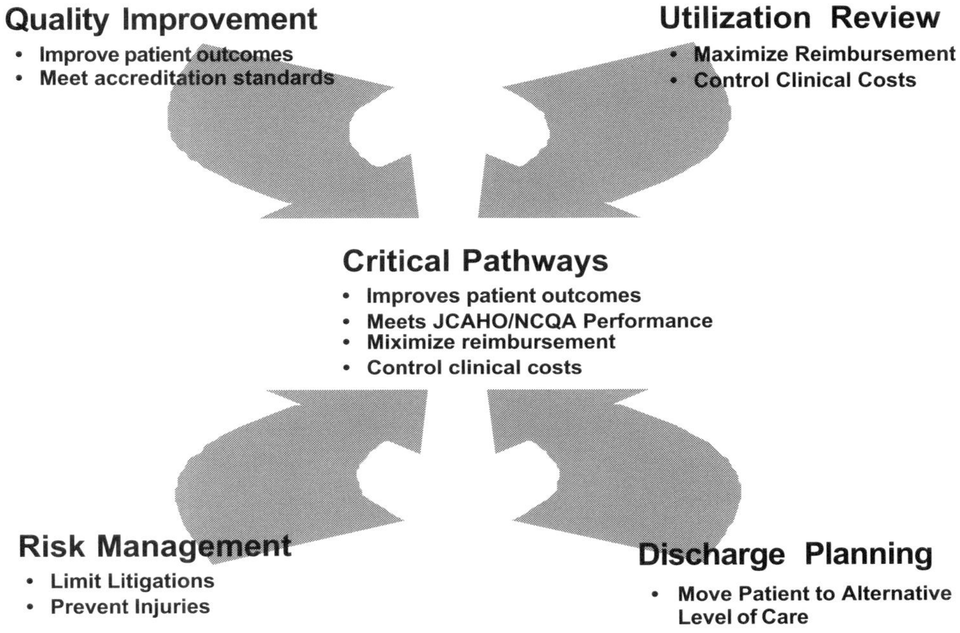

Quality Improvement
- Improve patient outcomes
- Meet accreditation standards

Utilization Review
- Maximize Reimbursement
- Control Clinical Costs

Critical Pathways
- Improves patient outcomes
- Meets JCAHO/NCQA Performance
- Miximize reimbursement
- Control clinical costs

Risk Management
- Limit Litigations
- Prevent Injuries

Discharge Planning
- Move Patient to Alternative Level of Care

Reengineering Principles

Before exploring how to reengineer current monitoring processes, some basic reengineering principles must be understood:

- Fundamental processes are reengineered, not departments
- Reengineering occurs from the top down
- Several tasks are combined into one process
- Work needs to be performed *when* it makes the most sense
- Work needs to be performed *where* it makes the most sense
- Processes have multiple versions

Each of these basic principles will be explained further in the following sections.

Focus on Redesigning Processes

The first reengineering principle is to focus on fundamental processes rather than a department or other organizational unit. **By focusing on processes, jobs, people and organizational structures experience dramatic changes.** For example, if an organization focuses on reengineering the quality management department, then only incremental improvements can be made because the quality management department is responsible for only part of the monitoring process. However, if an organization focuses on reengineering the patient care monitoring process, then dramatic changes can be realized by all departments and services which conduct patient care monitoring.

Focus Reengineering on Fundamental Patient Care Review Processes

- **Current Process**
  - **Department Specific**
  - **Administrative Task Specific**
- **Reengineered Process**
  - **Obtaining Payment**
  - **Obtaining Accreditation**
- **Identify Fundamental Processes**
  - **What must be done?**
  - **Why do we do what we do at all?**

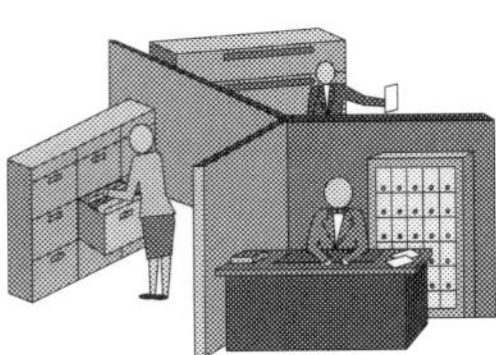

Functional departments
Fragmented processes

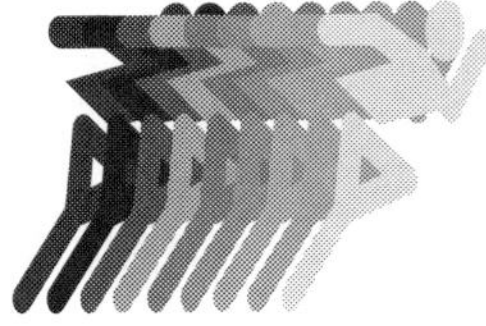

Processes have a beginning and an end

By focusing on patient care review processes instead of who does the work, we can recognize processes which are common to all departments or functions. The common activities performed by all patient review departments include:

- Finding cases for review
- Reviewing current clinical care using pre-established criteria

- Measuring the outcomes
- Investigating unacceptable variances or events
- Analyzing individual cases and aggregated data
- Communicating findings

Reengineer from the Top Down

Reengineering can never happen without top management support. There are two reasons for this axiom. One is that middle management and front-line employees lack the broad perspective that reengineering demands. The second is reengineering inevitably will cross organizational boundaries and require upper management authority to make changes.

To accomplish reengineering, there needs to be a senior executive leader who can act as visionary and motivator. This leader is self-nominated and self-appointed rather than assigned the responsibility. The reason leadership can not be assigned is because it is difficult to mandate a person to have a vision. The reengineering leader must:

- Articulate a vision of the "new" organization and standards
- Induce others to translate the vision into reality
- Create an environment conducive to reengineering
- Inspire others with a sense of purpose and mission

Reengineering Needs Top Management Involvement

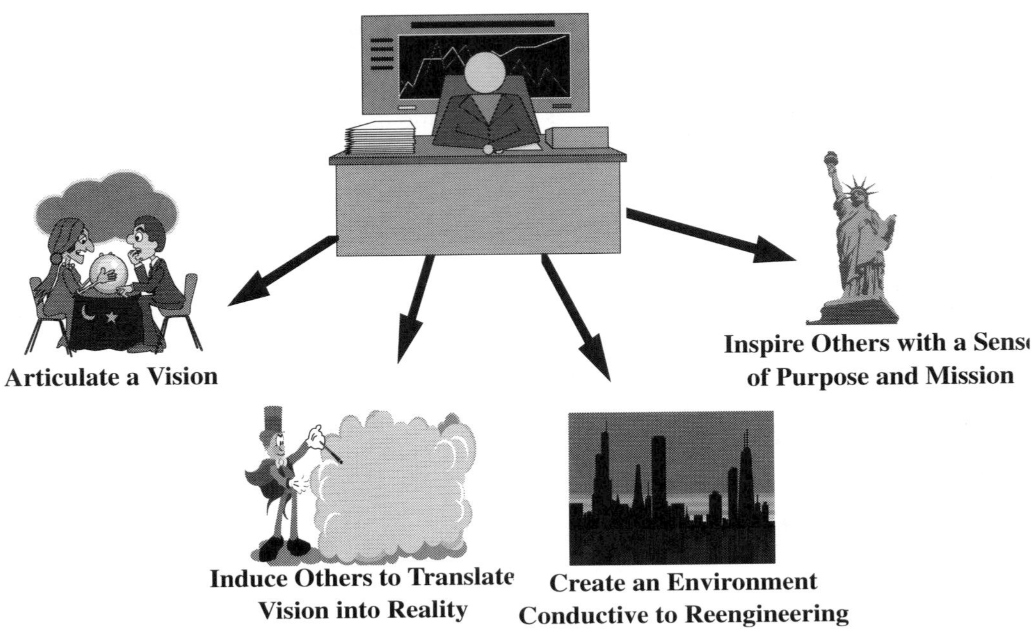

The reengineering leader can demonstrate leadership through signals, symbols and systems. Signals are explicit messages that the leader sends to the organization about reengineering: what it means, why we are doing it, how we are going about it and what it will take. Symbols are actions that the leader performs to reinforce the content of the signals, to demonstrate that he or she lives by his or her words: assigning the company's "best and brightest" to reengineering teams, rejecting design proposals that promise only incremental improvement, and removing managers and staff who block the reengineering effort. The leader also needs to use management systems to reinforce the reengineering message.

Combine Several Tasks into One Job

The most fundamental principle of reengineering is the integration and compression of fragmented activities into one process. To apply this principle, organizations need to compress responsibilities for the various steps in a process and assign it to one person. This person will become the case worker and is responsible for an end-to-end process. This scenario can work for the obtainment of payment process, where one person can be responsible for certifying the patient's insurance, moving the patient through the health care system and following-up on denied claims.

Many processes in health care cannot be integrated and assigned to one person because of the level of knowledge and skills required to perform many of the tasks. In this instance, a case team can be organized to perform the required process. **A case team** is a group of people who have among them the required skills. A patient focused unit is an example of a case team. **Case team members**, who previously were located in different departments, can be brought together into a single unit and given total responsibility for patient care. By integrating workers into teams, fewer people are involved, and the integrated process will be easier to control and monitor. Also, administrative overhead should be reduced. Another benefit of reengineering is that decision-making is part of the real work and not a separate function. This results in fewer delays, better customer response and greater empowerment of workers.

If a process is so complex or dispersed in such a way that integrating them for a single person or even a small team is impossible, a single point of contact needs to be designated. This person is called **a case manager** and acts as a buffer between the still complex process and the customer. The case manager behaves with the customer as if he or she were responsible for performing the entire process, even though that is really not the case. To be able to answer the customer's questions and solve customer problems, the case manager needs access to all the information systems that the people actually performing the process use and the ability to contact others with questions and requests for further assistance when necessary. Case managers need to be "empowered" customer service representatives.

Combine Serveral Tasks into One Job

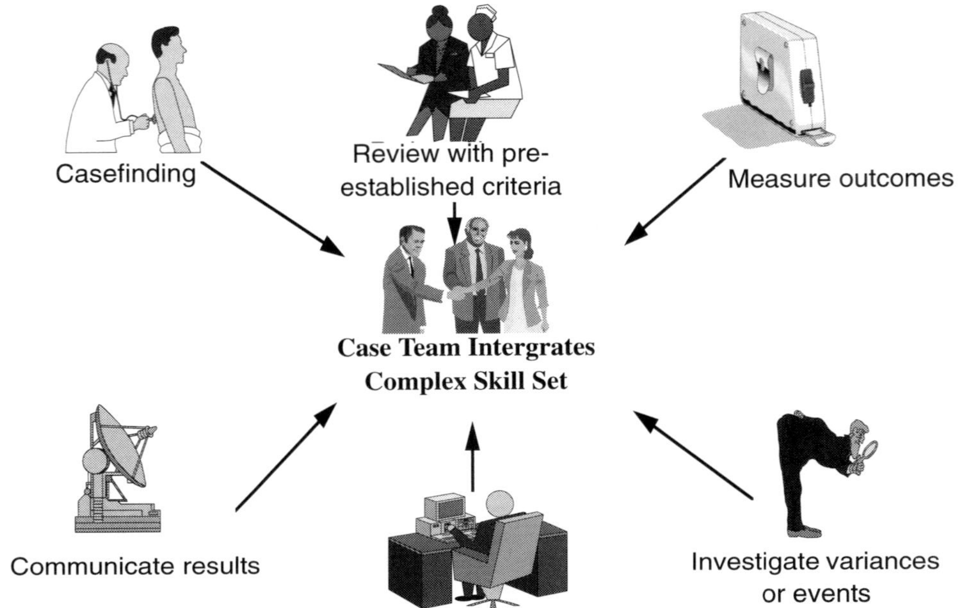

Perform Work When It Makes the Most Sense

Since reengineering integrates the process which is performed by a person or a team of people working closely together, work is freed from linear sequencing and the natural priority in the work can be used rather than the artificial one introduced by linearity. In reengineering, work is structured by what needs to follow what. "Delinearizing" processes speeds them up in two ways. One is the ability to get tasks done simultaneously, and the second is the reduction of elapsed time between early and late steps of a process. For example:

> When a patient is admitted to a facility, a demographic information sheet is entered into the computer by an admission clerk. This sheet is printed and placed in the patient's medical record. To start the utilization review process, many hospitals make a copy of the face sheet and send it to the utilization review department. The assigned staff takes the sheet and looks in the computer to determine if the patient has already been discharged. If the patient is still an inpatient, an initial utilization review is conducted. In a reengineered process, as soon as the admission clerk is has entered the patient name, reason for admission and insurance information, an e-mail message would be sent to the utilization review department. This would

eliminate waiting for the physical delivery of the face sheet and having to verify the patient's status.

Perform Work When and Where It Makes the Most Sense

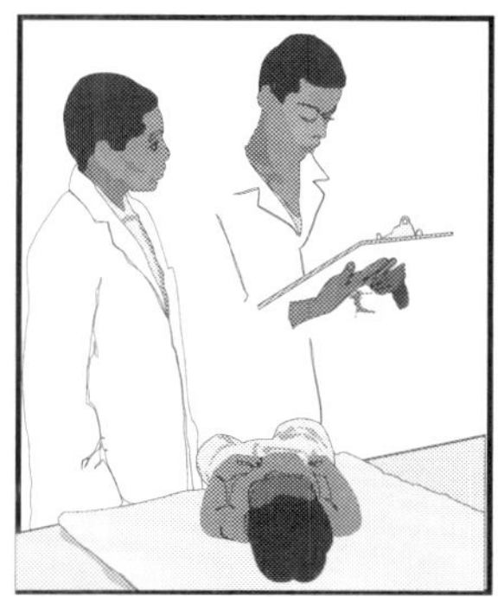

- **Perform Work When It Makes the Most Sense**
  - **Steps can be performed simultaneously**
  - **Flexibility eliminates elapse time**

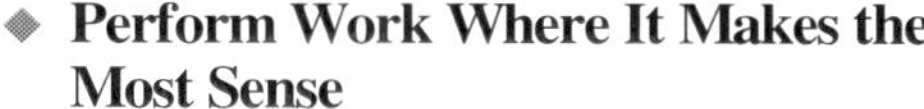

- **Perform Work Where It Makes the Most Sense**
  - **Processes are centered around patients, payers and accrediting agencies (instead of around specialists)**
  - **Sometimes suppliers and customers will perform some or all of the process**

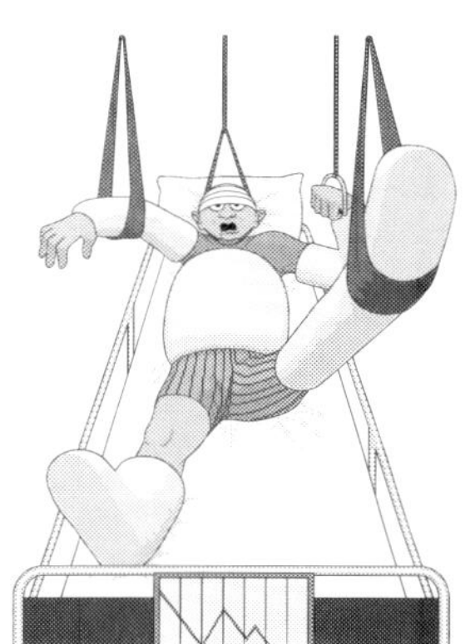

Perform Work Where It Makes the Most Sense

By shifting work across organizational boundaries, it can be performed more efficiently and with less overhead. **Traditionally work has been organized around a specialist instead of around the process that the specialist is trying to support.** For example, hospitals are frequently organized into departments. If a patient needs to receive care from the radiology, rehabilitation and respiratory therapy departments, the patient needs to be transported to each department. Through reengineering, services can be organized around the patient.

This principle can be applied to quality and resource management professionals by looking at where they perform most of their activities. Efficiency can be enhanced if the quality and resource management staff are decentralized among patient care areas.

Patient Care Review Needs a Combination of Centralization and Decentralization

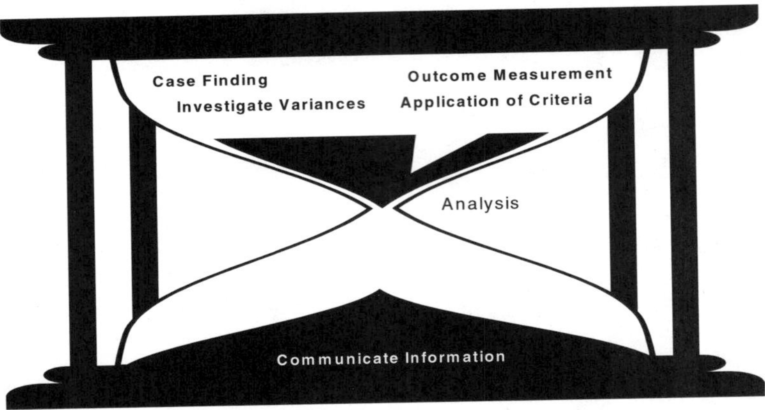

Processes Have Multiple Versions

A characteristic of reengineered processes is the end of standardization. To meet the demands of customers, we need multiple versions of the same process, each one tuned to the requirement of the patient it serves. For example, the process of taking care of a patient is very similar, and all patients need to be assessed and receive treatment. However, the type of assessments and treatments required for patient experiencing an acute myocardial infarction is very different from the requirements of a patient having a baby. Therefore, processes with multiple versions or pathways usually begin with a "triage" step to determine which version works best in a given situation. Simple triage needs to be based on some preestablished thresholds, which will facilitate a patient being admitted to the right process.

Processes Have Multiple Versions

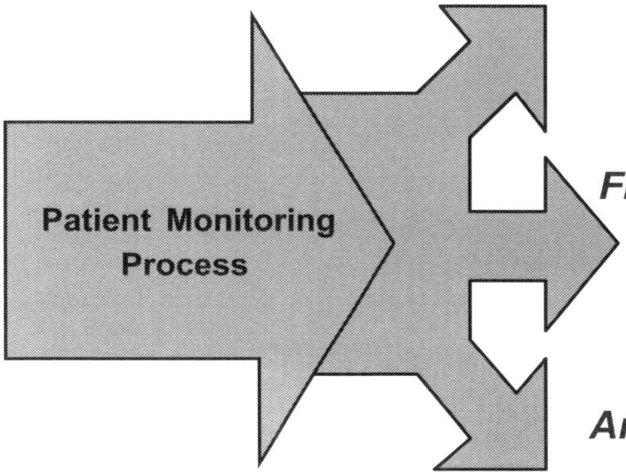

Congestive Heart Failure Pathway

- Case Selection Criteria includes SI
- Medication Usage Data
- Blood Usage Evaluation
- Department Specific PI
- Cardio-vascular IMS Outcome
- Measurements

Fractured Hip Pathway

- Case Selection Criteria includes SI
- Surgical Case Review
- Drug Usage Evaluation
- Blood Usage Evaluation
- Department Specific PI

Antepartal Care Pathway

- Case Selection Criteria includes SI
- Surgical Case Review
- Medication Usage Data
- Blood Usage Evaluation
- Department Specific PI
- OB IMS Outcome Measurements

Role of Information Technology in Reengineering

One thing to remember about reengineering is that it cannot happen in an organization that will not change the way it thinks about information technology. Information technology is an essential enabler of reengineering, though it must be used carefully in that context. Merely installing computers in an organization does not cause it to be reengineered. In fact, misuse of automation can block reengineering if it is used to reinforce old ways of thinking and existing behavior patterns.

"How can we use new technological capabilities to do things that we are not already doing?" One of the hardest parts of reengineering is recognizing the new, unfamiliar capabilities of technologies. This ability to recognize the power of modern information technology and to visualize its applications requires inductive thinking–the ability to first recognize a powerful solution and then seek the problems it might solve.

An important function information technology plays in reengineering is its ability to disrupt rules about how the work is conducted. For example, the belief that only specialists can perform complex work can be changed by the implementation of expert systems which enable generalists to do expert work. Another important function of information technology is the ability to make data simultaneously available to a wide range of people in many places. This accessibility to data breaks the restrictions placed on processes that have been dependent on the availability of a single file folder or medical record.

Role of Information Technology in Reengineering

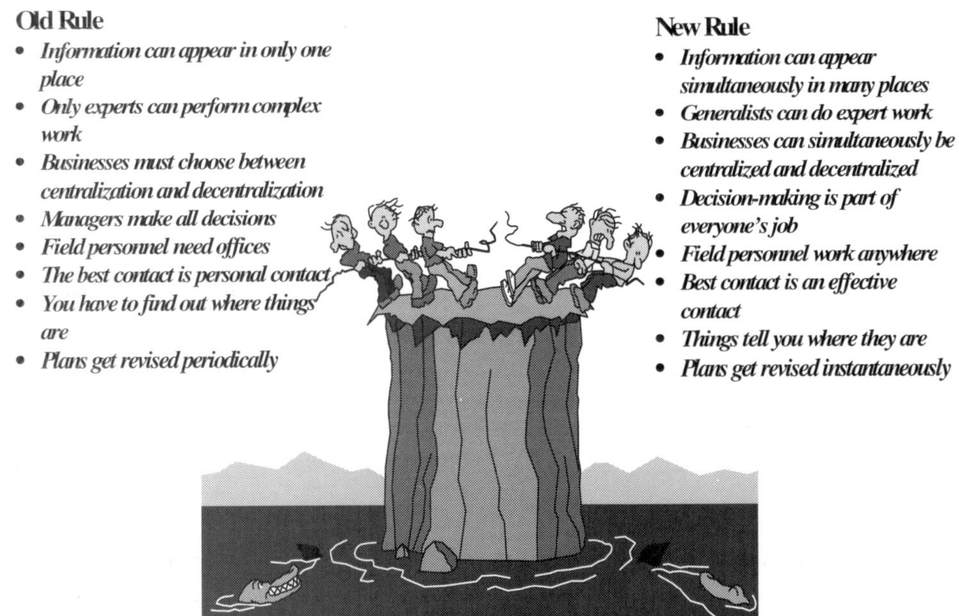

Case for Action

After a process is selected for reengineering, a case for action needs to be developed. This case for action communicates where we are, why we can't stay here and what we need to become. These messages are important to convey because people need a compelling reason for change.

There are five main parts to a case for action:

- Summary of the current situation and what is happening
- The problems with continuing the status quo
- Marketplace demands
- Explanation of why the current methods are unable to meet needs
- Cost of inaction

The case for action should be brief, no more than five to ten pages, and blunt. Here is an example of a case for action related to reengineering patient care review activities at Hospital Anywhere:

- We are unable to meet the need of clinicians, administrators and outside agencies for accurate, timely and meaningful data. We are spending 75 percent of our time collecting data and only 10 percent of our time converting it into information. This only leaves a total of 15 percent of our time to communicate information, provide education and manage quality projects.

- With the changes in the accreditation process, the increase in capitated funding and customers' increasing demand for accountability and cost-containment, we will be unable to meet the need.

- Our current method of conducting data collection causes duplication of effort, excessive workload and frustration. This will continue since data collection is fragmented and decentralized.

- We have strong competitive and economic incentives to move as quickly as possible toward an integrated data collection process. This will result in reducing the amount of time spent on data collection to 10 percent. Allowing time to meet the demands of staff, physicians and outside agencies for information, training and quality initiatives. We will be able to convert our image from a necessary evil to a vital information support.

- If we do not make this conversion, then we will lack the flexibility to meet changing regulations and standards, and information needed for negotiating managed care contracts will be unavailable. This can result in non-accreditation and reduction in revenues.

Vision Statement

Once a case for action is developed a vision statement needs to be communicated. This statement describes how the organization is going to operate and outlines the kind of results expected from the reengineering effort. It will:

- Outline the kinds of results expected
- Contain the qualitative and quantitative goals
- State which process actually needs work
- Provide a yard stick for measuring the progress of reengineering

This vision statement is different from the vision statements that are frequently the results of management retreats. This vision statement focuses on operations, establishes measurable objectives and may change the basis for competition in the industry.

The case for action and vision statements need to be used together because one gets people moving and the other indicates the direction. It is the leader's personal responsibility to articulate and communicate these key messages.

Reengineering Process

There is more than one way to reengineer a process. However, there are certain guidelines which have been proven useful in reengineering. These guidelines include:

- Redesigning is done best in teams
- The time between the beginning of reengineering and the initiation of the reengineered process should not exceed one year
- Start with desired results and work backwards
- Change a process, don't fix it
- Focus on processes
- Consider everything associated with the process being redesigned (job designs, organization structures, management systems, etc.)
- Expect disruption: if nothing is disrupted then no change has occurred
- Use people's values and beliefs in reengineering
- Demand dramatic results

- Eliminate all constraints on the definition of the problem and the scope of the reengineering effort
- Ignore existing corporate cultures and management attitudes
- Assign someone who understands reengineering to lead the effort
- Supply adequate resources
- Reengineering needs to be the top priority
- Plan the implementation carefully

2

Implementation of Critical Pathways

Introduction

Once a critical pathway has been developed, it is actualized through an implementation process. This process is the method an organization uses to promote pathway acceptance, modify current clinical practices and utilize the available infrastructure. To formulate a realistic implementation process, the oversight and pathway team members should collaborate to:

- Manage pathway implementation
- Develop support mechanisms
- Provide staff education

This chapter will focus on the components required to initiate and maintain critical pathways in an organization. Pathway advocates need to remember that pathway implementation, like pathway development, is a multi-disciplinary and collaborative effort rather than a one person assignment.

Manage Pathway Implementation

To begin the implementation process, pathway team members need to identify what tasks need to be accomplished for "rolling out" the developed critical pathway. Usually these tasks consist of:

- Conducting a "pilot test"

- Obtaining ratification or endorsement of the pathway
- Developing standardized recording and documentation forms
- Preparing patient education materials
- Establishing pathway guidelines and instructions
- Providing staff education
- Evaluating pathway effectiveness

How and when these activities are accomplished depends on the resources available, the intent of the pathway and the degree of resistance to change. By identifying what needs to be done and formulating a schedule for performing these tasks, team members can successfully implement a pathway.

To develop and manage critical pathway implementation effectively, the pathway team needs to understand several principles of project management. These principles include:

- Implementation activities need to be divided into small tasks. Each task should be small enough that it can be accomplished within five working days. The ability to divide a large project into manageable tasks will increase the potential for success and prevent the feeling of being overwhelmed.
- The higher a person is in the organization's hierarchy, the longer the duration is between task assignments. For example, a staff nurse can be assigned a specific task every week while the unit director's assignments should be every other week and so forth.
- Projects that fall behind can be put back on schedule through one of four methods: changing the timeframe, reducing the scope, assigning more resources or sacrificing quality.
- Tasks within a project need to be assigned to a specific person with the expertise to accomplish the task.
- Relationships between tasks need to be identified and assignments sequenced to ensure smooth implementation.
- Resources need to be identified to complete the assigned tasks. Resources include time, money, people, education and materials.
- Tasks should be linked to specific dates for completion.

Shown on the next few pages is a generic implementation plan which serves as a basis for developing pathway specific project plans.

TABLE 1. Pathway Implementation Plan

Project Activity	Start Date	End Date	Assignment	Resource
I. Pilot Study of Pathway				
a. Provide education for staff involved in pilot study				
b. Initiate pilot study of ten cases				
c. Collect data				
d. Analyze data				
e. Revise pathway based on pilot study				
II. Ratification of Pathway				
a.				
b.				
c.				
d.				
e.				
III. Develop Pathway Communication Materials				
a. Create medical record forms				
b. Create pathway monitoring forms				
c. Type pathway forms				
d. Print forms				
IV. Pre-printed Physician Orders				
a. Create medical record forms				
b. Type orders				
c. Distribute orders				
V. Develop Instructions and Define Terms				
a. Review current pathway policy				
b. Create specific instructions				
c. Define key terms which are unique to this pathway				
d. Prepare instructions				

TABLE 1. Pathway Implementation Plan

Project Activity	Start Date	End Date	Assignment	Resource
VI. Develop Patient Education Materials				
a. Identify pathway elements for patient pathway				
b. Create patient education materi-als				
c. Type final materials				
d. Print patient education materials				
VII. Staff Education about Path-way				
a. Design staff education program				
b. Prepare educational materials				
c. Schedule inservices				
d.				
e.				
f.				
VIII. Report Pathway Results				
a. One month report				
b. Two month report				
c. Three month report				
IX. Identify Triggers for Revisions				
X. Disband and Celebrate				

Pathway Implementation Strategies

During the past several years, many organizations have attempted to implement critical pathways with varying degrees of success. The three most common problems which arise during pathway implementation are:

- Lack of clinician acceptance
- Inconsistent application of pathways
- Inability to manage pathway data

We will spend the rest of this section exploring possible causes and strategies for dealing with the issues mentioned above.

Lack of Clinician Acceptance

One of the most common problems found by pathway advocates is the lack of clinician acceptance. There are several reasons for this situation. The most common reason is the lack of early participation with the pathway process. Many organizations make the mistake of creating a pathway and then announcing to physicians and other affected clinicians that it **must** be used. This promotes a feeling of being out of control or helpless.

To promote acceptance, physicians and other involved clinicians need to be involved from the very beginning of the pathway process. This will allow advocates to address the reasons for resistance and incorporate suggestions into the developing pathway.

It is imperative for pathway advocates to recognize that **pathways cannot be mandated**. This attitude is important because people will frequently resist being changed but will change if the idea was their own.

Inconsistent Application of Pathways

The second most common problem is the inconsistency of applying pathways. This inconsistency results from lack of staff education, sporadic distribution of support mechanisms and a lack of a recognized pathway process. For example, a patient is placed on a total hip replacement pathway, and on the second day of care, an agency nurse takes care of the patient. Because she is unfamiliar with the content of the pathway, several of the pathway elements were not performed, thus the pathway is inconsistently applied.

This issue can be addressed by educating staff regarding pathway content, how to use pathways and staff responsibilities. This education needs to be ongoing and included in the orientation of new staff. Another strategy is to make someone accountable for coordinating patient care according to the pathway.

To prevent sporadic distribution, organizations can disseminate all pathway packets from a central location such as the admission or emergency departments. Patients then arrive on a patient unit or outpatient location with their own pathway packet. Another strategy can be used if an organization is automated. Pathway forms can be computer generated and made available throughout the organization via computer networks.

Inability to Manage Pathway Data

The third most common problem with implementing pathways is an organization's inability to manage pathway data. This problem arises when organizations have not clearly identified the pathway goals and critical elements. **To prevent this problem pathway teams need to take time to identify outcome measurements and critical interventions.** This will prevent an organization from being overwhelmed with collecting clinical information and assigning variances to aspects of care which do not impact desired patient goals. Most organizations that are overwhelmed with pathway data are doing clinical pathways and eventually give up measuring care.

Another strategy is to do random sampling of cases which have the potential of being placed on the pathway. This will allow clinicians to validate their pathway and keep the process manageable.

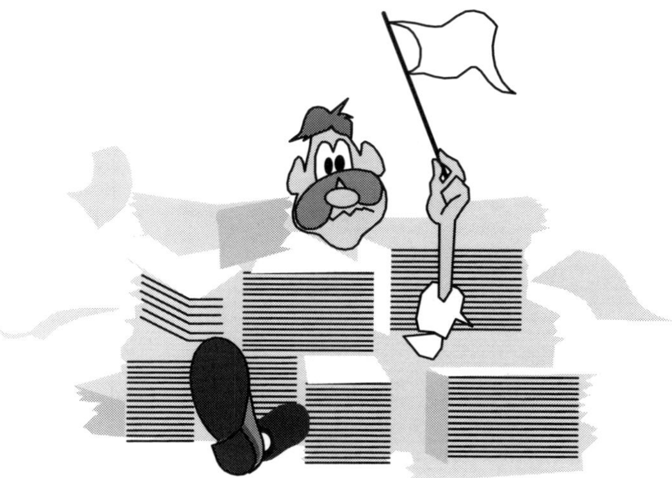

One of the newest and best solutions for managing pathway data is to automate the pathway process. If current information management hardware and software can't support collection and analysis of pathway data, pathway processes will be labor intensive and very difficult to implement successfully.

To automate the process, clinicians may need a combination of software products which can interface with each other to capture data at the point of care, identify pathway variances, analyze process and outcome data and compare pathway and non-pathway care. At the current time the only products that can accomplish these activities are Pathbuilder™ and CaseMaster™.

Development of Support Mechanisms

A key component of successful implementation is the availability of support mechanisms. These mechanisms include:

- Pathway guidelines or procedures
- Documentation and recording systems
- Patient education materials
- Product and service delivery systems

These support mechanisms ensure consistent use of the developed pathway, facilitate recording of pathway interventions and patient response, promote patient participation and promote collaboration among treatment team members.

Guidelines or Procedures

Implementation guidelines or procedures are developed to ensure consistent application of pathways. These guidelines need to outline staff responsibilities, define key terminology and pathway procedures. They generally take the form of instruction sheets or organizational policies and procedures. An example of a critical pathway policy and procedure is provided in Appendix A.

Staff Responsibilities

Implementation guidelines must clearly define the nature and scope of staff responsibilities and apportion tasks among individuals and groups. Decisions made during the "assignment of responsibilities" phase of implementation will impact the scope of assignments. A responsibility statement looks like this:

> **The Attending Physician** is responsible for initiating and discontinuing a critical pathway. The attending physician will serve as the case leader for all care. If a variance is noted in the **medical care**, the attending physician is responsible for documenting the reason for this variance and, if appropriate, taking action to return the patient to the pathway.

Staff roles and responsibilities, commonly defined in a pathway policy and procedure, include:

- Oversight Committee
- Case Coordinator or Clinical Case Manager

- Medical Executive Committee
- Caregiver
- Clinical Departments
- Medical Staff Departments

Key Pathway Definitions

To promote consistent use and documentation of critical pathway elements, key terms need to be defined in the guidelines. These terms may include *critical pathway, day of care, point of service* and *variance*. By clearly defining key words, consistency of care and documentation are enhanced.

For example, the term *day of care* can be correctly defined as either "the care provided during a specific date," or "care provided within a 24 hour period of time, beginning at the moment the patient enters the health care organization." However, if the term is not pre-defined, each clinician will interpret it differently and perform the scheduled interventions differently.

TABLE 2. Sample Pathway Definitions

Pathway Terms	Definition
Day 1	The span of time from the moment a patient initially makes contact with the organization to midnight on the same date. This includes the initial time spent in the emergency department.
Visit 1	The first home service visit after the initial intake visit.
Case Coordinator	The staff member assigned responsibility for coordinating the patient's care according to the pathway. This varies according to the point in service and type of patient care provided.
Case Leader	The attending physician at the time when care is delivered.
Variance	Any deviation from the pathway schedule of a critical intervention.
System Variance	A deviation from the critical pathway caused by a breakdown in (or unavailability of) an organization's delivery systems or by equipment failure.
Patient Variance	A deviation from the critical pathway caused by a change in the patient's condition, unavailability or actions.
Practitioner Variance	A deviation from the pathway caused by an omission or commission of a caregiver.
Practitioner	Any individual who provides clinical care to patients. This term is used synonymously with caregiver and clinician. Physicians, nurses and social workers (among others) are all practitioners.

Pathway Procedures

Probably the most important part of critical pathway guidelines is the outline of critical pathway procedures. These procedures describe the steps required to implement, use and document a critical pathway. Minimally, critical pathway procedures need to address:

- Initiation of a critical pathway
- Utilization of a pathway to provide patient care
- Documentation of a pathway
- Documentation of variances
- Discontinuation of a pathway
- Pathway revision process

It may be helpful to clinicians to have a flow chart which will outline the clinical pathway process. This will enable them to see the entire process at one time.

Critical Pathway Clinical Process

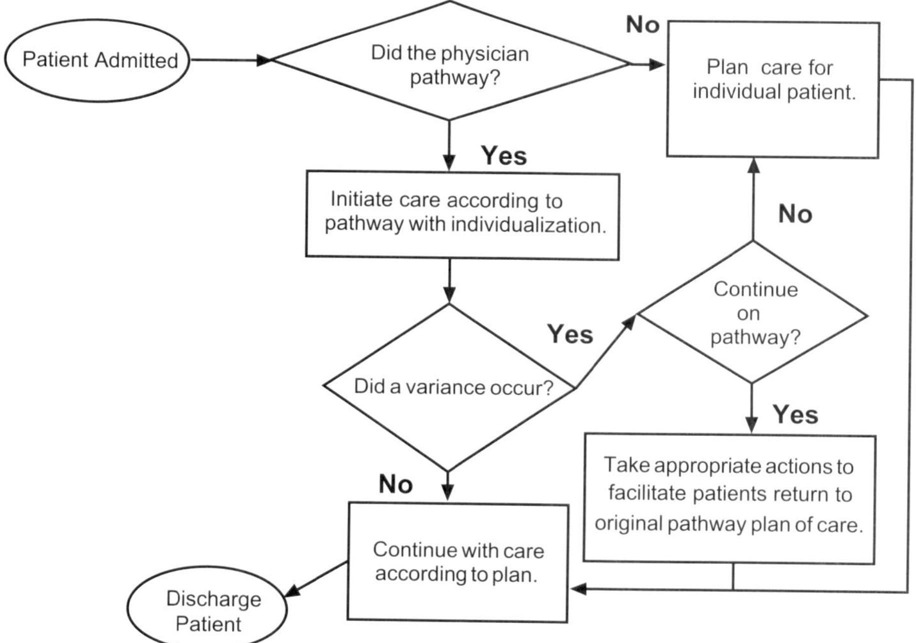

Once critical pathway guidelines are developed, they can form the basis for critical pathway orientation and just-in-time education.

Documentation and Recording Systems

Many clinicians fear that pathways will increase the amount of required documentation. Before we start exploring possible documentation systems for pathways, we need to revisit current processes and requirements.

There are three basic types of information which are recorded in the medical record. These types are:

- **Routine information:** This information is independent of the patient's condition but is dependent on the organization's policies and procedures and/or outside agency standards and regulations. Examples of routine information are vital signs, amount of food eaten, patient bath, initial nursing assessment, history and physical, etc.
- **Critical information:** This information is based on the patient's condition and includes data about critical assessments and interventions. This information relates to the elements on the critical pathway.
- **Optional information:** This information is based on a caregiver's values or secondary conditions, such as co-morbidities and pre-existing conditions. For example, a patient who is being treated for congestive heart failure may also be a diabetic. However, the patient's diabetes is stable and does not require treatment.

By understanding the type of information which make up current documentation, we can start developing a documentation system which can streamline and standardize the recording of essential information.

Creating Individualized Care From Pathways: Implementing Macro Solutions For Micro Problems

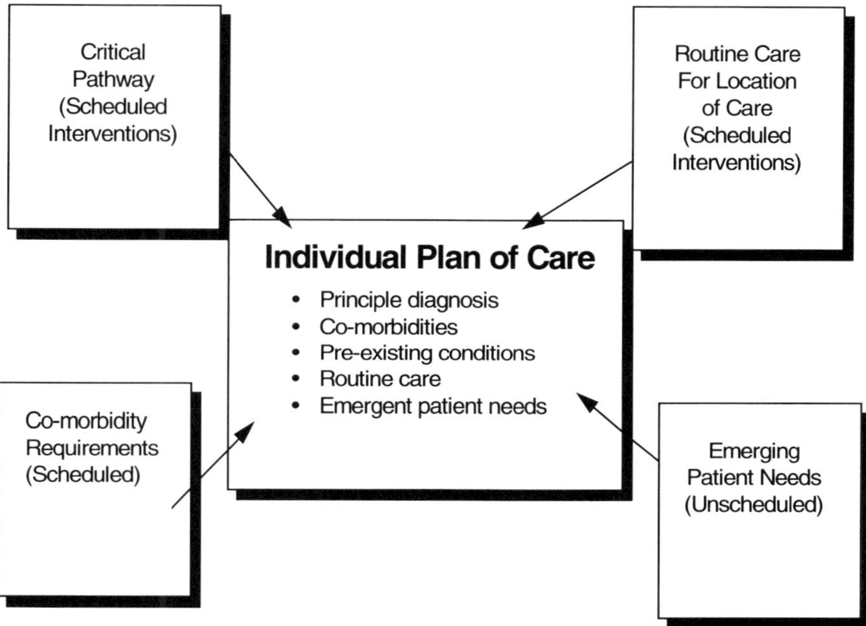

There are several basic guidelines which need to be followed when developing any documentation system. Documentation should:

- Support practitioners' decisions, not make the decisions.
- Match the facility's basic documentation philosophy (e.g., focused, problem oriented or narrative charting).
- Allow for concise recording of patient assessments as well as interventions.
- Record only information regarding the patient not highlight system and practitioner variances. The word variance should not appear in the medical record.
- Meet current medical record standards and regulations.
- Focus on eliminating or preventing duplication of effort.
- Facilitate protection from malpractice litigation.

To create a realistic documentation system, we will need to review the current documentation system to identify its strengths and weaknesses. From this assessment clinicians will need to decide the best way to consolidate, revise or replace different forms to promote fast and easy documentation. For example, we may consolidate all patient education documentation into a single multi-disciplinary educational record.

Creating a Documentation System

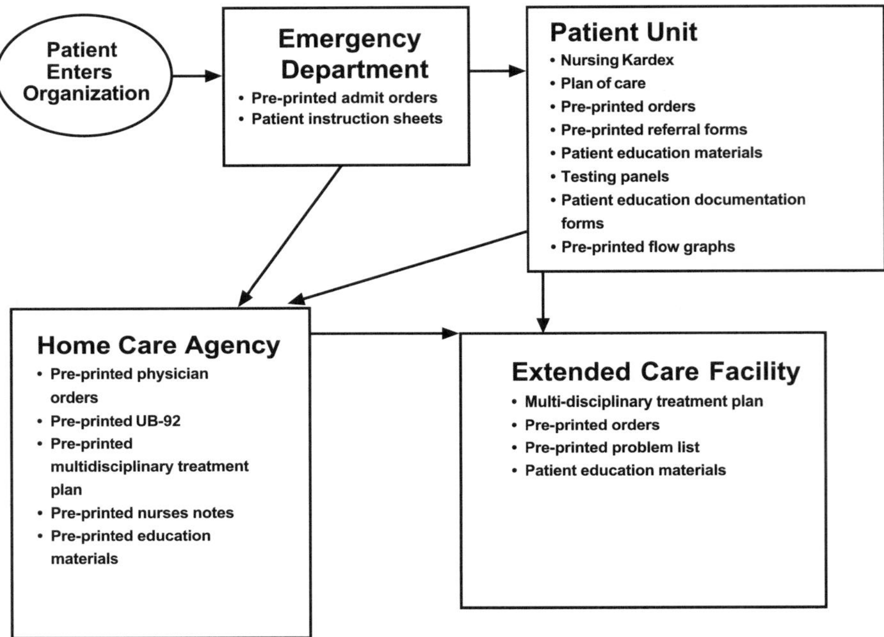

It is important to develop a documentation system which will support both pathway and non-pathway care. This will enable clinicians to use one documentation system for all patient care. This will decrease possible confusion and increase the likelihood of consistent pathway application. Typical documentation forms which may be considered for revision are:

- Pre-printed physician orders
- Patient education records
- Multi-disciplinary plan of care
- Referral forms and consultation requests
- Progress notes
- Nursing kardex (hard copy or electronic)

These are the basic mechanisms for communicating information between clinical disciplines and recording vital patient information.

There are two basic approaches for documenting pathways. One approach consists of placing a copy of the critical pathway in the medical record as a plan of care which will be used as a point of reference for physician orders and documenting interventions. The second approach is to use pathways as the basis for documentation. Each of these systems will be explored further.

Pathway Reference Guides

A documentation system for pathways can use the pathway as a guide for providing care. The pathway form may be a permanent or temporary part of a patient's medical record.

Pathway reference guides enable clinicians to continue to use current medical record forms, controlling printing costs as well. However, an issue remains regarding, where to place the guide to facilitate consistent use by caregivers. Additionally, because the pathway is not integrated into the documentation system, there is a higher risk of practitioners forgetting about the pathway. An example of a pathway guide is shown below.

The operational issues which must be addressed if an organization decides to use a pathway guide are:

- Will it be a permanent or temporary part of the medical record?
- Where will it be placed to facilitate consistent use by caregivers?
- How will it be used to communicate completion of pathway interventions?
- What current support mechanisms can be replaced by the pathway guide?

Clinicians and administrators need to identify the mechanisms currently used for communication between practitioners, disciplines and departments. Among others, these mechanisms may include the use of a patient kardex, a multi-disciplinary treatment plan or a computer generated plan of care. An organization should take into account these existing documentation processes in deciding whether the pathway guide should be a permanent or temporary part of the medical record.

If the pathway guide replaces a temporary communication form such as the patient kardex then the guide should be only temporary. If the pathway guide is used as the multi-disciplinary treatment plan, as required in long-term care, homecare and psychiatric care, then the pathway guide should be a permanent part of the medical record.

Based on whether the pathway guide is temporary or permanent, clinicians can then decide how the guide will be used to communicate completion of pathway elements. For example, if the pathway guide is used as a patient kardex, it can serve as a checklist for expected interventions, similar to a surgical checklist. If the guide is used as a multi-disciplinary treatment plan, only changes in the plan of care will be documented on the guide.

A critical operational issue is where the guide should be placed to facilitate consistent utilization by caregivers. For ease of use, there may be more than one copy of the pathway guide used at one time. This can lead to confusion and/or redundancy. An organization should decide which copy of the pathway guide is the principle copy and designate an owner for that copy. A suggested approach is to give the assigned case coordinator responsibility for keeping the principle copy current.

Hospital Anywhere - CHF - Systolic Dysfunction

	Hour 0-2	Day 1	Day 2	Day 3	Day 4	Day 5
PATIENT ASSESS-MENT	_Blood pressure (Q30 minutes)	_Weight (daily before breakfast using same scales)	_Weight (daily before breakfast using same scales)	_Weight (daily before breakfast using same scales)	_Weight (daily before breakfast using same scales)	_Weight (daily before breakfast using same scales)
	_Breath sounds (every shift)	_Blood pressure (with TPR Q4H)	_Blood pressure (with TPR Q4H)	_Blood pressure (with TPR Q4H)	_Blood pressure (with TPR Q4H)	_Blood pressure (with TPR Q4H)
	_Peripheral edema	_Breath sounds (every shift)	_Breath sounds (every shift)	_Breath sounds (every shift)	_Breath sounds (every shift)	_Breath sounds (every shift)
		_Peripheral edema (every shift)	_Peripheral edema (every shift)	_Peripheral edema (every shift)	_Peripheral edema (every shift)	_Peripheral edema (every shift)
DIAG-NOSTIC TESTS	_ECG	_Arterial blood gases (if currently on oxygen)	_Electrolytes	_Arterial blood gases (if currently on oxygen)	_Arterial blood gases (if currently on oxygen)	
	_Chest x-ray	_Continuous cardiac monitoring	_Echocardiogram (if echo, MUGA or catheterization not previously performed)	_Continuous cardiac monitoring (continue if cardiac arrhythmias present)	_Continuous cardiac monitoring (continue if cardiac arrhythmias present)	
	_Electrolytes		_Arterial blood gases (if currently on oxygen)			

Hospital Anywhere - CHF - Systolic Dysfunction

	_Digitalis blood level (if currently taking digoxin)		_Continuous cardiac monitoring (continue if cardiac arrhythmias present)			
	_Complete blood count					
	_Cardiac profile					
	_Arterial blood gases					
	_Continuous cardiac monitoring					
TREATMENTS	_Oxygen therapy	_Oxygen therapy (if oxygen saturation level below 90%)	_Oxygen therapy (if oxygen saturation level below 90%)	_Oxygen therapy (if oxygen saturation level below 90%)	_Oxygen therapy (if oxygen saturation level below 90%)	
MEDICATION USAGE	_Diuretics	_Angiotensin converting enzyme inhibitors	_Angiotensin converting enzyme inhibitors	_Angiotensin converting enzyme inhibitors	_Angiotensin converting enzyme inhibitors	_Angiotensin converting enzyme inhibitors
	_Vasodilators	_Diuretics	_Diuretics	_Diuretics	_Diuretics	_Diuretics
		_Vasodilators	_Vasodilators	_Vasodilators	_Vasodilators	_Vasodilators
NUTRITION AND FLUIDS	_Intravenous fluids	_Intravenous fluids	_Intravenous fluids	_Low-sodium diet	_Low-sodium diet	_Low-sodium diet
		_Low sodium diet	_Low sodium diet			
CONTINUITY OF CARE		_Discharge plan				

Hospital Anywhere - CHF - Systolic Dysfunction

PATIENT EDUCA-TION		_About dis-ease condi-tion		_About dis-ease condi-tion	_Medication education: cardiac med-ication (writ-ten instructions)	_What is expected of patient (review post hospital care)
		_'What is expected of patient (give patient path-way)		_About low sodium diet		

Pathway Documentation Forms

A second approach is to provide pre-printed forms such as physician orders and progress notes for each pathway. This approach is more directive and emphasizes standardized assessments and interventions.

The advantages of using pre-printed forms are constant daily reminders of expected assessments and interventions, rapid documentation and easy identification of pathway variances. Disadvantages include higher costs associated with producing forms and the possibility the forms may not be completed. By having a blank or incomplete form in a medical record, questions are more apt to arise about non-compliance with standards of practice and care.

If an organization decides to develop medical record forms to support critical pathways, it needs to consider what type of information will be documented, who will record the information and where the forms will be used.

Progress notes and other medical record forms can be modified to reflect the elements of a critical pathway. These modifications can include developing multi-disciplinary progress notes, which reflect the timing of pathway interventions, patient assessments and pathway variances. It is important that clinicians record only patient-centered information and not practitioner or system variances in the medical record. Examples of pre-printed physician progress notes, nurses' notes and a multi-disciplinary progress note are shown on the following pages.

When pathway advocates are developing forms for physician orders, they need to remember that the physician still retains legal responsibility for the care of the patient. Because of this responsibility, organizations can develop pre-printed physician orders, but not automatic standing orders. Pre-printed orders differ from standing orders because they facilitate rapid physician ordering, support professional judgment, reinforce the physician's responsibility for patient care and are legal.

Besides developing pre-printed physician orders and progress notes, organizations may consider creating pre-printed consultation and laboratory forms and radiology requisition panels. All of these efforts can improve efficiency and facilitate timely scheduling of interventions.

Day 1:	Day 2:	Day 3:
Patient Assessments: Weight before breakfast: Breath sounds: N: ____ Breath sounds: D: ____ Breath sounds: E: ____ Peripheral edema: N: ____ Peripheral edema: D: ____ Peripheral edema: E: ____ TPR: Q4th: (See vital signs sheet)	**Patient Assessments:** Weight before breakfast: Breath sounds: N: ____ Breath sounds: D: ____ Breath sounds: E: ____ Peripheral edema: N: ____ Peripheral edema: D: ____ Peripheral edema: E: ____ TPR: Q4th: (See vital signs sheet)	**Patient Assessments:** Weight before breakfast: Breath sounds: N: ____ Breath sounds: D: ____ Breath sounds: E: ____ Peripheral edema: N: ____ Peripheral edema: D: ____ Peripheral edema: E: ____ TPR: Q4th: (See vital signs sheet)
Treatments: Oxygen therapy:	**Treatments:** Oxygen therapy:	**Treatments:** Oxygen therapy:
Nutrition and Fluids: IV fluids:	**Nutrition and Fluids:** IV fluids:	**Nutrition and Fluids:** IV fluids:
Continuity of Care: Discharge planning assessment: No further planning needed: See progress note below:	**Continuity of Care:** Discharge planning assessment:	**Continuity of Care:**
Patient Education: (Pt. Ed. Form) About disease condition: What is expected of patient:	**Patient Education:**	**Patient Education: (Pt. Ed. Form)** About disease condition: Low-sodium diet:

Caregiver's name and initials: ____________________

Date/Time	Progress Note

		Hospital Anywhere
Date	Time	Physician Orders (SYSTOLIC DYSFUNCTION HEART FAILURE)
		PATIENT ASSESSMENT
		- Patient Weights (Use the same scales and weigh before breakfast) - (Day 1, Day 3 thru Day ___)
		- Vital signs with B/P QID
		DIAGNOSTIC TESTS
		- ECG - (Hour 0-2)
		- Chest X-ray - (Hour 0-2)
		- Cardiac monitoring - (Hour 0-2 thru Day 4)
		– Echocardiogram (If echo, MUGA or catheterization not previously performed) - (Day 2)
		- Electrolytes - (Hour 0-2, Day 2, Day 4)
		- Cardiac Profile - (Hour 0-2)
		- Digitalis level (if taking digitalis prior to admission) - (Hour 0-2)
		MEDICATION USAGE
		- Diuretic therapy (________mg_____q .) - Hour 0-2 thru Day 5)
		- Vasodilators (________mg______) (Hour 0-2 thru Day 5)
		- Anticoagulant therapy (___________q___) - (Day 1 thru Day 5)
		- Analgesic:
		- Hypnotic:
		NUTRITION AND FLUIDS
		- Low-sodium diet - (day 1 thru day 5)
		CONTINUITY OF CARE
		- Discharge planning - (Day 1)
		- Dietary referral - (Day 1)
		ACTIVITY
		- Up as tolerated

Hospital Anywhere - Systolic Dysfunction Heart Failure

	Hour 0-2	**Day 1**	**Day 2**	**Day 3**	**Day 4**	**Day 5**
PATIENT ASSESS-MENT	_Blood pressure	_Blood pressure (QID)	_Blood pressure	_Blood pressure	_Blood pressure	_Blood pressure
	_Breath sounds	_Breath sounds	_Breath sounds (every shift)	_Breath sounds	_Breath sounds	_Breath sounds
		_Patient weights (Use the same scales and weigh before breakfast)	_Patient weights (Use the same scales and weigh before breakfast)	_Patient weights (Use the same scales and weigh before breakfast)	_Patient weights (Use the same scales and weigh before breakfast)	_Patient weights (Use the same scales and weigh before breakfast)
		_Peripheral edema assess-ment	_Peripheral edema assess-ment	_Peripheral edema assess-ment	_Peripheral edema assess-ment	_Peripheral edema assess-ment
DIAG-NOSTIC TESTS	_Blood gases	_Cardiac monitoring	_Cardiac monitoring	_Cardiac monitoring	_Cardiac monitoring	
	_ECG	_Cardiac monitoring	_Echocardio gram (if echo, MUGA or catheteriza-tion not pre-viously performed)		_Electrolytes	
	_Chest X-ray		_Electrolytes			
	_CBC					
	_Cardiac Monitoring					
	_Electrolytes					
	_Cardiac Profile					
	_Digitalis Level (if tak-ing digitalis prior to admission)					

Hospital Anywhere - Systolic Dysfunction Heart Failure

MEDICATION USAGE	_Diuretic therapy (________mg _____q .)	_Diuretic therapy (________mg _____q .)	_Diuretic therapy (________mg _____q .)	_Diuretic therapy (________mg _____q .)	_Diuretic therapy (________mg _____q .)	_Diuretic therapy (________mg _____q .)
	_Vasodilators (________mg _____)	_Digoxin	_Digoxin	_Digoxin	_Digoxin	_Digoxin
		_Vasodilators (________ mg _____)	_Vasodilators (________ mg _____)	_Vasodilators (________ mg _____)	_Vasodilators (________ mg _____)	_Vasodilators (________ mg _____)
	_Anticoagulant Therapy (__________ q_____	_Anticoagulant Therapy (__________ q_____	_Anticoagulant Therapy (__________ q_____	_Anticoagulant Therapy (__________ q_____	_Anticoagulant Therapy (__________ q_____	_Anticoagulant Therapy (__________ q_____
NUTRITION AND FLUIDS		_Low-Sodium Diet	_Low-Sodium Diet	_Low-Sodium Diet	_Low-Sodium Diet	_Low-Sodium Diet
PATIENT EDUCATION		_Disease Condition	_Low-sodium Diet (dietary counseling)	_Exercises	_Medication Education	
CONTINUITY OF CARE		_Discharge Planning				
		_Dietary Referral				

Multidisciplinary Education Record

Instructed Key: P = Patient F = Family/Significant other

Outcome Key: S = Understanding or performs successfully

R = Needs reinforcement or repeat demonstration

U = Unable to comprehend or perform

E = See comments/follow-up

Patient Education Assessment Result:

Learning Disabilities: None Other

Language: English Other

Special considerations:

Patient Education Topic	Date	In-struct	Date	In-struct	Date	In-struct	Date	In-struct
	Ini-tials	Out-comes	Ini-tials	Out-comes	Ini-tials	Out-comes	Ini-tials	Out comes
Low-Sodium Diet								
Needed:____ Not needed:____								
Medication Education: Diuretic Therapy								
Needed:____ Not needed:____								
Medication Education: Digoxin Therapy								
Needed:____ Not needed:____								
Medication Education:								
Needed:____ Not needed:____								
Disease Condition								

Patient Education Topic	Date	In-struct	Date	In-struct	Date	In-struct	Date	In-struct
	Ini-tials	Out-comes	Ini-tials	Out-comes	Ini-tials	Out-comes	Ini-tials	Out comes
Needed:____ Not needed:____								
Exercises								
Needed:____ Not needed:____								

Name								
Initials								
Department								

Patient Education Materials

Patient education conveys two types of information. First, patients must be given information about self-care activities, such as proper transfer techniques, insulin administration and how to do dressing changes. Secondly, patients must be made aware of the critical pathway, the expectations for their role in the pathway process and the expected outcomes. By acquiring this information, patients are able to:

- Collaborate with caregivers to actively participate in their own care
- Understand and reach expected patient goals
- Make preparations for post pathway care

There are several concepts to keep in mind while developing educational materials for patients. These concepts are:

- Information should be stated in layman's terms to enhance patient understanding

- Most patient education material needs to be developed for a fourth grade level
- Critical pathway elements should be described from the patient's perspective
- A pathway is only a guide for care and not an authoritative source
- Educational materials need to be relevant, short and simple
- Interactive learning materials are better than one-way materials

Patient Education Example for Total Hip Replacement Patient Pathway

Before Admisson

You will have a physical exam by your family doctor. Two weeks before surgery you will have a blood test and may donate some blood. This blood will be available for your own use. It will be given only if needed. You will need to attend a pre-operative class at the hospital before your surgery. Please call: 555-1000 to schedule your class and arrange transportation. At this class you will learn what exercises you will need to do after surgery. You will meet the nursing staff, the discharge planner, physical therapist and case coordinator.

Day of Surgery

You will be taken from the admission office to the Same Day Surgery Department. Prior to surgery, you will have a tube called an intravenous tube placed in your vein. This tube will be used to give you liquids and medicine. After surgery you will have a large dressing on your hip. You may have a drain in your hip to help reduce swelling. **You will need to do your ankle pumps, arm strengthening and bed exercises, as well as use the triflow bottles every hour while awake.** You will have a tube in your arm which will be used to give you fluids. You will have a blood test to determine if you will need blood. You will be given an antibiotic to prevent any infection. If you are having pain, please request pain medication. This will help you move better after surgery.

If you cannot urinate within 8 hours after surgery, the nurse may place a tube in your bladder to help you pass water.

First Day After Surgery

The bandage on your hip will be changed during the morning. You will go to the physical therapy department twice a day to learn how to use crutches or a walker. **You will need to continue your ankle pumps, arm strengthening and bed exercises, as well as use the triflow bottles every hour while awake.** If you are able to eat and drink at least half of every meal without vomiting, then the tube in your arm will be removed.

On the first day after surgery you will have a blood test in the morning to determine if you will need to receive any blood.

Product and Service Delivery System

Because pathways standardize patient care, organizations can begin to manage delivery services better. For example, if a patient is placed on a total hip replacement pathway, central supply knows at the beginning of the pathway what supplies are required. They can provide them in a timely manner directly to the patient's bedside. This will reduce the amount of time a caregiver spends looking for supplies and recording supply charges. Other delivery systems which can be streamlined and changed to support pathways are:

- Medication delivery systems
- Diagnostic test scheduling and processing
- Ancillary service schedules

Pathways can be Used as a Basis to Plan and Deliver Patient Care Services

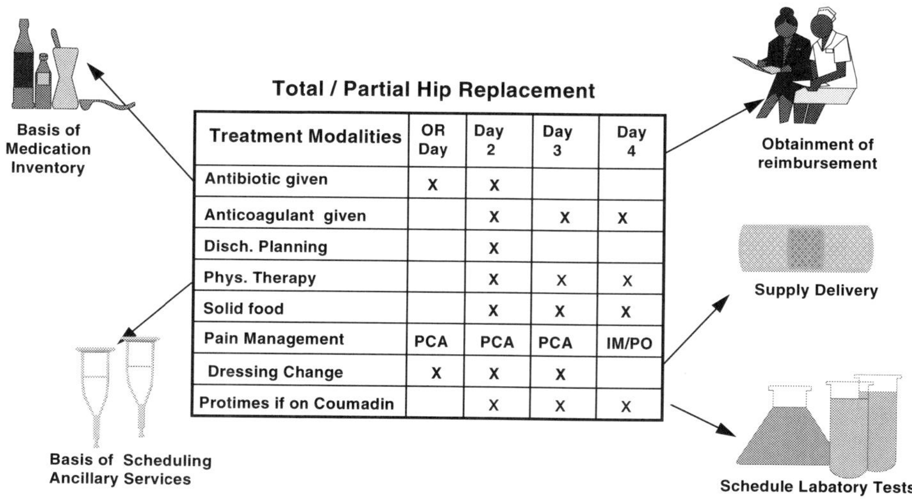

Treatment Modalities	OR Day	Day 2	Day 3	Day 4
Antibiotic given	X	X		
Anticoagulant given		X	X	X
Disch. Planning		X		
Phys. Therapy		X	X	X
Solid food		X	X	X
Pain Management	PCA	PCA	PCA	IM/PO
Dressing Change	X	X	X	
Protimes if on Coumadin		X	X	X

Provision of Staff Education

One of the key ingredients for a successful critical pathway implementation is to provide appropriate, timely and relevant staff education. There are three basic types of education associated with implementing critical pathways. They are:

- Orientation
- Skill building
- Just-in-time education

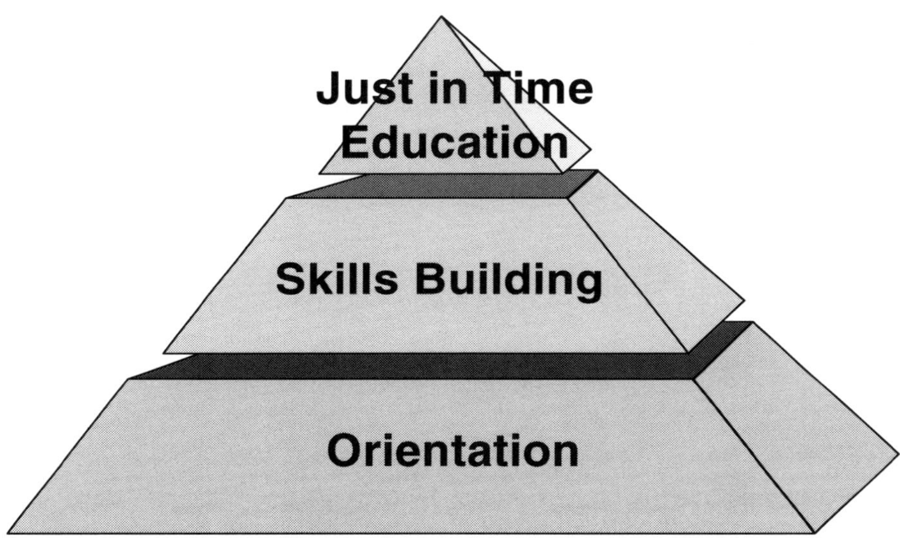

Orientation to Critical Pathways

Orientation provides general information about how to use critical pathways as well as the expected impact. General information about the organization's pathway process should be shared with clinicians and administrative staff. This will promote "unfreezing" of the staff's perception about how pathways will be used and will initiate the "move" to the new way of providing care. Pathway advocates will need to:

- Illustrate the need for critical pathways by displaying data
- Explain the goals of the pathway process
- Present pathway guidelines, policies and procedures
- Explain pathway responsibilities
- Address questions and concerns

Pre-established forums such as department, patient unit, committee and multi-disciplinary treatment planning meetings are good venues for communicating this information. Special meetings, videos and programs can also be used to provide this orientation.

By openly communicating the reason for the pathways, how they will be used and what impact can be expected, pathway advocates promote acceptance by clinicians who were not involved in the development process. These staff members then become aware of the need for change and can provide input into the implementation process. As a result, they become part of the "team."

In summary, orientation will prepare clinicians to use critical pathways by outlining the organization's philosophy for pathways, and reducing anxiety about practice changes.

Skill Building Education

During the critical pathway development and implementation process, clinicians may identify the need for new knowledge, skills or abilities. Skill building education to meet these needs can be provided through in-service, continuing education programs or formal education classes. This type of education could, for example, include instructions about new procedures, medications or equipment usage.

Skill building education generates an important link between clinical quality improvement activities and the knowledge and skills needed to perform assigned responsibilities. This linkage provides a means to improve organizational performance, successfully implement pathways and meet the Joint Commission's standards for "Orientation Training and Education of Staff."

Related to skill building education is proficiency-based orientation for new staff. This proficiency system can use the pathway skills to develop organization or unit-based proficiency checklists. The checklist shown below is a sample of a pediatric asthma proficiency checklist.

TABLE 3. Pediatric Asthma Nursing Proficiency

Proficiency Skill	Date of Demonstrated Proficiency	Name of Certifier
Breath Sounds Assessment		
Dyspnea Level Assessment		
Peak Flow Meter Use		
Nebulizer Therapy		
Moderate Asthma Pathway Usage		

Just-in-Time Education

As critical pathways are being implemented, education of the involved clinicians needs to occur regarding the day-to-day application of a particular critical pathway. This education covers what is contained in a specific critical pathway, how to document the care given and how to handle variations from the pathway.

Clinician instruction should occur just prior to initial use of the pathway. "Just-in-time" education is recommended since adults retain information longer if new knowledge can be immediately applied.

In addition to the initial in-service on a new critical pathway, just-in-time education should be presented to clinicians when:

- Questions arise about specific critical pathways
- Reasons for a pathway variance are unclear
- New staff members are added

The individual responsible for this education can be another peer, a case coordinator, a clinical nurse specialist, a nurse manager or the pathway coordinator.

Organizations can facilitate successful implementation of critical pathways by providing appropriate staff education. Educational programs provide a mechanism for modifying clinical practice, improving consistency of care, enhancing staff competency and promoting compliance with pathways.

Implementation Exercise: Applying Pathway Policies and Procedures

1. Using the Critical Pathway Policy Statement in the first column, decide how to handle the situation described in the second column. State your group's decision and any policy changes required in the third column. (15 minutes)

TABLE 4.

Policy Statements	Situation	Decisions and Policy Recommendations
Critical pathways are considered a plan of care which can be ordered by the attending physician. If an existing critical pathway is not ordered, the physician will develop a plan of care within the first 24 hours of admission.	A patient has been admitted to the medical center with a diagnosis of bacterial pneumonia. The doctor did not order the bacterial pneumonia pathway, but states in progress notes, "Patient has secondary diagnoses of C.O.P.D., diabetes mellitus type II, dehydration and hypertension. Due to patient's severity and age of 92 years, pathway will not be used."	
When the patient is transferred from one unit to another, the RN assuming care for the patient will receive a report on the patient's progress along the critical pathway, any variances, and actions taken.	A patient who has been on the major depression pathway for the past two days, suddenly becomes cyanotic and complains of chest pain. This patient is transferred to the Medical Intensive Care Unit for possible myocardial infarction.	
The critical path will be used as a reference point for consultations between team members, during MD rounds and at patient care conferences.	It is now 3:00 p.m. and according to the pathway for total knee replacement the patient should have been seen by Physical Therapy today for total knee rehabilitation.	

TABLE 4.

Policy Statements	Situation	Decisions and Policy Recommendations
The critical pathway case coordination form is a temporary part of the medical record. After discharge it will be sent to the Quality/ Resource Department for completion and analysis.	A patient has been discharged from the 3-West telemetry unit after being on the elective PTCA pathway. When the record arrives in the Medical Record Department for abstraction a case coordination form is found.	
A patient can be removed from the pathway when the patient deviates significantly from the pathway. This decision must be made by the attending physician. To discontinue a pathway, the time, date and reason for discontinuation must be recorded on the case coordination form.	It is 1:00 a.m. and a patient on the acute myocardial infarction suddenly experiences acute chest pain and has a cardiac arrest. A code is called and the patient is transferred to Coronary Care Unit.	
When a patient on a pathway is discharged from one facility to another level of care, the pathway plan for aftercare will be documented on the discharge summary and reported to the receiving agency.	A patient on the COPD homecare critical pathway is admitted to a local hospital with bacterial pneumonia. The primary care nurse was at the patient's house at the time of the transfer to the hospital.	

3

Measurement of Results

Introduction

After a critical pathway has been implemented, the impact on patient care needs to be measured. This is done to *assess pathway compliance*, *discover opportunities for improvement* and *evaluate goal attainment*. Clinicians must establish a monitoring system which collects pathway information, manages individual cases and analyzes pathway data.

Collection of Pathway Information

To manage pathways effectively, organizations need to establish a means for collecting, analyzing and distributing relevant data. To begin, we need to assign responsibility for managing individual cases and collecting data, identify information to be collected and plan data collection.

Assignment of Responsibilities

There has been much discussion about who should be responsible for collecting and managing critical pathways. In some organizations, a member of the nursing staff is responsible for providing care and collecting pathway data. In another organization, a utilization reviewer is responsible for coordinating pathway cases and collecting pathway data. In a third organization, a social worker is responsible for performing discharge planning and collecting pathway data. In all three organizations, the assigned person is called a **case manager**. Despite the popularity of the term case manager, there is no universal consensus about who qualifies as a case manager and what responsibilities are encompassed in this role.

For our purposes, we have decided that true case management is best performed by a team of people with a variety of skills. This team consists of a care manager, case manager and information specialist. Each of these roles and responsibilities will be discussed in the subsequent paragraphs.

We have designated the term **care manager** to refer to the individual assigned the task of managing the clinical care of the patient according to a specific critical pathway. This role does not encompass data collection or deal with the financial aspects of the case. Staff members who demonstrate clinical expertise should be considered for the care management functions.

The range of responsibilities for a care manager includes:

- Collaborating with other treatment team members to facilitate appropriate application of pathways
- Coordinating care within a health care organization
- Providing just-in-time education to other staff members regarding patient care
- Documenting patient care

The care manager role may or may not have direct patient care responsibilities and can be assigned to a nurse, social worker, physical therapist or pharmacist depending on the type of patient receiving care. By separating the clinical care manager from the financial and data collection responsibilities, an existing position such as a charge nurse, clinical nurse specialist or clinical pharmacist can fulfill the role without increasing the number of employees needed.

An individual who is responsible for coordinating discharge planning, performing utilization reviews, conducting pathway monitoring and investigating variances is a **case manager.**

The range of responsibilities for the case manager includes:

- Monitoring application of pathways
- Investigating the reasons for variances
- Facilitating continuity of care within the health care system
- Documenting variances and corrective actions
- Collecting pathway data

If a position is assigned both care and case management responsibilities, then it would qualify as a **case coordinator**. This role truly coordinates the clinical, financial and informational aspects of the case.

The final member of the case management team is an **information specialist**. This role requires skill in study design, managing and analyzing clinical and financial data. The role is responsible for:

- Aggregating clinical data
- Performing statistical analysis of clinical and variance data
- Computing cost benefit analysis
- Preparing information for clinician analysis
- Serving as a consultant to pathway teams and clinical departments regarding study design and data analysis.

A key organizational issue concern is who should serve as the care and case managers. The assignment of these responsibilities varies between organizations and levels of care, but should be determined by which person has the knowledge, skills and experience to best perform each function. The table shown below highlights possible candidates for each position based on generalized assumptions about the skills present in the candidate groups.

TABLE 5.

Level of Care	Care Manager	Case Manager
Acute Care Facility	Clinical Nurse Specialist or Primary Care Nurses, Clinical Pharmacists	Quality / Resource Management Staff or Unit Manager
Psychiatric Facility or Unit	Primary Therapist or Nurse	Quality / Resources Management Staff or Unit Manager
Home Health Agency	Assigned Home Health Care Nurse	Case Manager or Director of Clinical Services
Rehabilitation	Physical Therapist or Occupational Therapist	Quality / Resource Management Staff
Outpatient Clinic	Patient	Nurse

Identification of Pathway Data

The final issue in developing a monitoring process involves which critical pathway information should be collected for analysis. It is advisable for organizations to collect information about individual pathway elements, the reasons for variance from the pathway and the outcomes of the pathway.

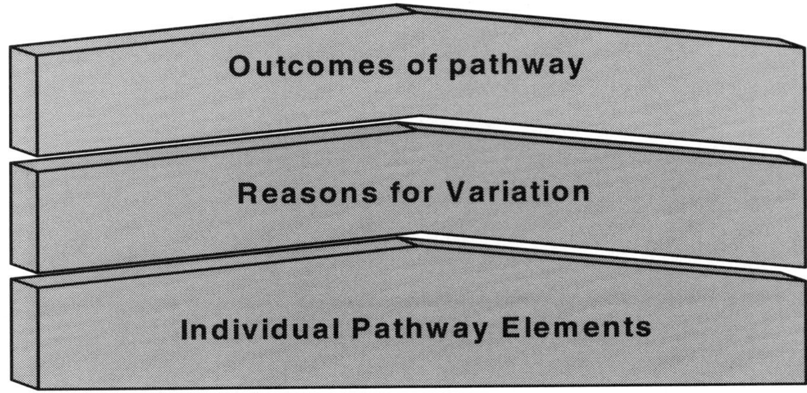

Measuring Individual Pathway Elements

Since clinicians are monitoring a critical pathway and not a clinical pathway, all elements are essential and should be monitored. By monitoring the presence or absence of each scheduled pathway assessment and intervention element, an organization can:

- Assess the stability of the patient care process
- Make refinements to the existing critical pathway
- Plan future staff education

Measuring Reasons for Variance

The second type of measurement relates to identifying the reasons for pathway variations. By investigating the reason for pathway deviations, areas for improvement can be identified and evidence can be accumulated to support new or existing continuous quality improvement efforts. The reasons for pathway deviation can be grouped into three categories:

- Patient issues
- Practitioner issues
- System issues

Variance Monitoring

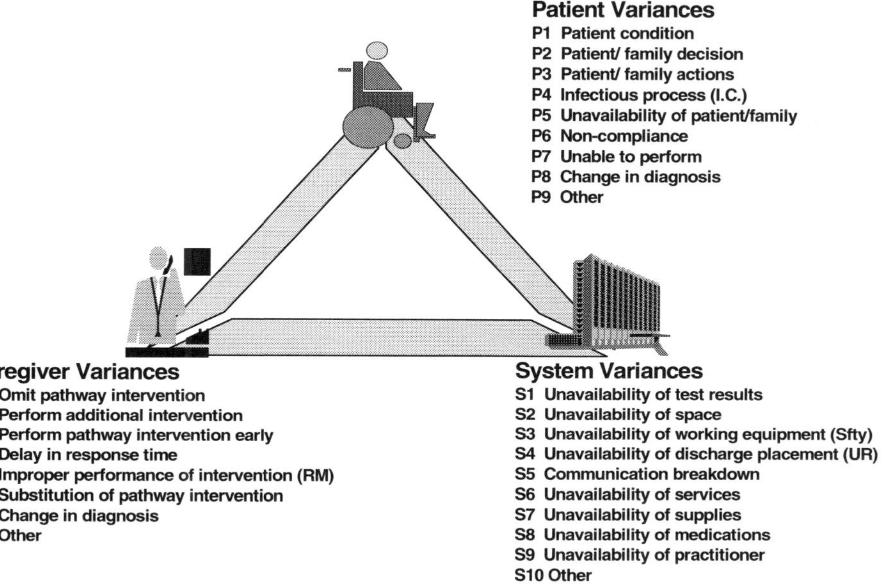

Patient variances can result from changes in a patient's condition along with patient (or family) decisions, actions and availability. Deviations caused by patient issues identify possible areas for pathway revisions and suggest potential population re-structuring for future pathway development.

The second type of variance is related to system issues. These include equipment failures, unavailability of services, products or equipment and breakdown in communication. Data from system issues can be used to determine projects for future continuous quality improvement teams.

The final type of pathway variance relates to practitioner issues. The term practitioner is used generically and means any caregiver, be that physician, nurse or other clinician. Practitioner variances arise from:

- Omission of a pathway element or changes in timing or duration of pathway interventions without providing a patient-centered reason or system variance for doing so
- Performing a pathway element incorrectly
- Substituting a similar type of action for a pathway element

Often practitioner variations are used to plan future staff education programs or to initiate peer review activities. However, they can also form the basis for pathway revisions if improved patient outcomes are achieved through non-conforming practices.

Those monitoring care need to remember to rule out system and patient variances prior to identifying a variance as a practitioner issue. The reason for this sequence is that critical pathways only address the critical elements of care. Additional elements may be required to provide optimal care.

Decision Model for Assigning Variances

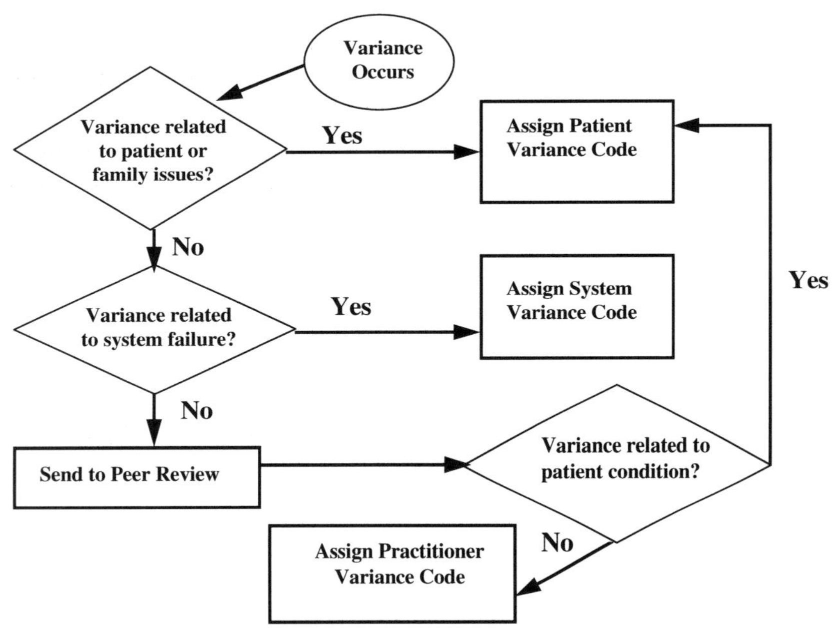

Developing a Variance Identification System

To create useful and relevant variance reason codes, clinicians should identify:

- Relevant categories of variance reasons. For example, patient, system and caregiver represent three possible variance categories.
- Types of variance reasons. For example, condition, decision, availability, action, knowledge and concomitance are all types of reasons.

- Operational definitions for each type of variance. For example, the operational definition for patient condition is "All pathway element variances which result from the patient not requiring the intervention, the intervention being contra-indicated or as a result of a co-morbidity."
- Questions which case managers can ask to validate appropriate assignment of variance reasons. For example, a clinician omitted a specific intervention on the pathway. This variance was classified as a caregiver omission. However, by asking "Does the caregiver have privileges to perform this intervention?" and "Was a caregiver available with the needed privileges?" Case managers can determine if this is really a caregiver variance or a system issue.

An important concept is that the complexity and specificity of a variance tracking system is dependent on the type of automation used for collecting and analyzing variance data. For example, if an organization is using a manual system for tracking variance reasons then the specificity of analysis is limited to the general types of variances with ancedotal comments. If an organization is automated then variances can be classified by both general and secondary levels of variance types. Table 6 outlines examples of variance types.

TABLE 6. Possible Variance Tracking

Variance Category	Type of Variance	Type of Variance Sub-group (Place in comments or sub-group if automated)	Validation Questions
Patient	Condition	• Contra-indicated • Co-morbidity • Does not require • Increase severity	
Patient	Decision	• Refuses • Requests • Postpones	

TABLE 6. Possible Variance Tracking

Variance Category	Type of Variance	Type of Variance Sub-group (Place in comments or sub-group if automated)	Validation Questions
Patient	Availability	• Late • Earlier • Not here	Was the patient informed about the schedule? If not, assign a System Communication variance code.
	Infection	• Community acquired • Nosocomial	
	Knowledge	• Able to demonstrate • Knowledge deficit • Need for repetition • Lack of readiness	
	Action	• Performs incorrectly • Refuses	
	Resources	• Financial support not available • Social support not available	
System	Diagnostic Testing	• Results not available • Results available earlier • Test not performed • Test results invalid	
	Equipment	• Doesn't exist • Non-functional • Unavailable • Able to use earlier	

TABLE 6. Possible Variance Tracking

Variance Category	Type of Variance	Type of Variance Subgroup (Place in comments or subgroup if automated)	Validation Questions
System	Services	• Not available • Doesn't exist • Available earlier	
	Supplies	• Not available • Damaged • Wrong supplies obtained	
	Medication	• Not available • Available earlier	
	Space	• Not available • Available later • Available earlier	
	Communication	• Message not sent • Receiver not available • Message unclear • Message not initiated	
	Community	• Resource not available • Available earlier	

TABLE 6. Possible Variance Tracking

Variance Category	Type of Variance	Type of Variance Sub-group (Place in comments or sub-group if automated)	Validation Questions
Caregiver	Knowledge	• Not in privileges (job description) • Unable to perform • Based on new standards • Based on external reference	Did the caregiver have privileges to perform this intervention? If not, was there a caregiver available with these privileges? If not, assign variance to "Services not available."
	Timing	• Delay response • Available earlier	Was the caregiver notified of need? If not, assign to "communication" variance.
	Preference	• Omitted • Additional interventions • Substitution • Duplicate same intervention	Did the patient require this intervention? If not, assign to "Patient Condition." Was the medication, supply or equipment available? If not, assign to correct "System Variance."
	Techniques	• Performed incorrectly • New technology • New method • Alternate techniques	

Measuring Patient Outcomes

Monitoring patient outcomes is the last type of critical pathway measurement. Outcome measurements can focus on the attainment of daily progress goals (if they were developed) and/or individual case outcomes. By aggregating the individual case outcomes, clinicians can measure the degree to which a critical pathway meets its intended purpose. Outcome measurements should reflect attainment of the pathway goals created during the pathway development phase.

Plan Data Collection

Once pathway management has been assigned, and data has been identified for collection, it is time to develop a plan for collecting and analyzing pathway data. The plan for data collection needs to guide the monitoring process by addressing operational issues such as the timing of data collection, what cases will be measured and how to handle variances.

Timing of Data Collection

Pathways can be monitored either retrospectively or concurrently. The resources needed to conduct the monitoring function include knowledgeable staff, accurate medical record coding information and sufficient time.

Concurrent monitoring is defined as reviewing the care provided to patients **during** an episode of care. It is the preferred method of review, though it is also more labor intensive and costly. Monitoring a critical pathway concurrently allows rapid correction of pathway deviations, provides the information required for insurance reviews and facilitates identification of system variance. The disadvantage of concurrent monitoring is the incompleteness of outcome data and the higher cost of monitoring.

Retrospective monitoring is defined as reviewing the care provided to patients **after** an episode of care is complete. This method of review allows the collection of all critical pathway data during a single review of the medical record. The advantages of retrospective monitoring include lower cost and the availability of complete patient care and practitioner information regarding accurate diagnoses, clinical interventions and outcomes. The disadvantages of retrospective review are delays in impacting care and difficulty in identifying system issues.

The information extracted during the pathway measurement process can be used in a multitude of ways. If measurements are conducted concurrently, the information can provide a basis for utilization reviews, infection control surveillance and interdisciplinary monitoring and evaluation. If measurements are conducted retrospectively, the information can be used to meet monitoring and evaluation requirements, such as drug usage evaluation, pertinence of medical records, surgical case reviews and interdisciplinary reviews.

Data Collection Process

Because critical pathways will provide the data for ongoing quality/ resource management monitoring, they should be applied to all cases which qualify for a pathway regardless of whether clinically the patient is placed on the pathway or not. The reason for this is to validate that the original assumptions made about pathway elements are true and to continually improve patient care.

Critical Pathway Monitoring Process

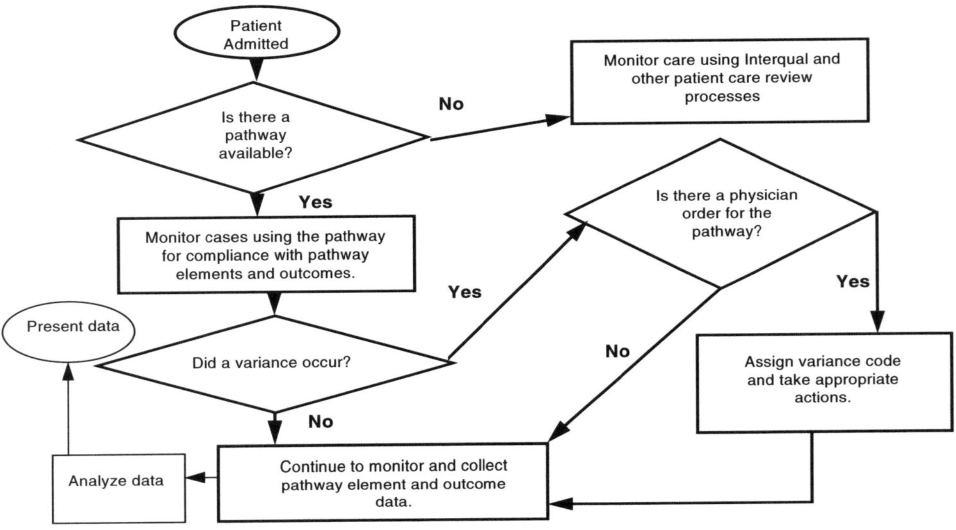

Manage Individual Cases

To efficiently and consistently collect critical pathway measurement data and to manage patients on critical pathways, a case management plan needs to be developed. This document serves as a critical pathway monitoring, utilization review and discharge planning form.

The case management plan contains information about critical pathway activities, the actions taken to promote pathway compliance, the reasons for deviations from the pathway and the outcome of the case. Additional information, such as discharge planning and insurance review information, may be recorded on the case management form if it lies within the case manager's responsibilities.

To ensure consistent use of the case management plan, explicit instructions need to be developed for both the management process and for filling out the form. These instructions can be included in the implementation guidelines or policies or they can be a separate instruction sheet or policy.

Issues to be addressed in the case management guidelines include:

- How to complete the form
- Definition of terms
- Decision rules
- What to do with the information when the form is complete

An example of these guidelines is found in Appendix A under Procedures, section D. A sample case management plan is shown on the next pages.

Analysis of Data

Once data has been collected for the established critical pathway, it needs to be analyzed so that continuous quality improvement occurs.

Clinicians frequently wonder what to do with critical pathway data. This information can be aggregated to:

- Identify process and outcome variations
- Provide insights into health care system breakdowns
- Compare actual practice with formulated goals

To accomplish critical pathway analysis, comparisons must be made among pathway elements, clinicians' performance, reasons for variations and patient outcomes.

EXAMPLE: Community-acquired Bacterial Pneumonia (Adult)

Allergies: Rm #:	Admit date:____ Discharge date:____ LOS:______ Nursing unit:_______ Diagnosis: bacterial pneumonia Procedure:_________________

Addressograph stamp

Aspects of Care	0-2 Hours	Day 1	Day 2	Day 3	Day 4
1. Assess-ments	1. V/S with B/P 2. Dyspnea level 3. Breath sounds 4. LOC 5. Skin color 6. Presence of cough	1. TPR every 4 hrs 3. Breath sounds q4h 4. LOC q4h 5. Skin color q4h 6. Cough q4h	1. TPR every 4 hrs 3. Breath sounds q4h 4. LOC q4h 5. Skin color q4h 6. Cough q4h	1. TPR every qid 3. Breath sounds qid 5. Skin color qid 6. Cough qid	1. TPR qid 3. Breath sounds q shift 5. Skin color q shift 6. Cough q shift
2. Diagnos-tic tests	1. Chest X-ray 2. Electro-lytes 3. CBC 4. Pulse ixim-etry or ABGs 5. Blood cul-ture qh X 2 prior to anti-biotic given 6. Sputum gram stain prior to anti-biotic 7. Sputum culture prior to antibiotic	4. Pulse oximetry or ABGs if on oxygen ther-apy	4. Pulse oximetry or ABGs if put on oxygen therapy	1. Chest X-ray 3. CBC 4. Pulse oximetry or ABGs if put on oxygen therapy	

Case Management Action Plan:

Instructions: Record the date of each variance from the pathway, the pathway element number, the variance code, corresponding actions, any additional comments and your initials in the appropriate space listed below. If no variances are noted in the case, check the box below **patient outcomes**.

Date	**Function of Care**	**Pathway Element**	**Timing of Var.**	**Var. Code**	**Action Code**	**Comments**	**Reviewers' Initials**

Return completed form to the Quality/Resource Management Department within 24 hours of patient discharge.

Pathway Data Collection Log

Pathway:____

Date	Pt. MR #	MD #	Pt Unit	Function of Care	Pathway Element	Timing of Var.	Variance Code	Action Code	Comments	Patient Outcomes		

Pathway Elements

Clinicians need to the analyze the proportion of cases complying with each critical pathway element. This analysis can be done longitudinally to show changes in the critical pathway process over time.

> For example, when a critical pathway is first implemented, the percentage of cases receiving ACE inhibitors is 20 percent. As time progresses, this percentage rises to 80 percent. This aggregated compliance data demonstrates the effectiveness of implementation efforts and the relevancy of the developed pathway element. If clinicians start to notice a trend in decreasing compliance rates for a specific data element, they may suspect a destabilization of the current process.

By using histograms and/or run charts to plot proportions of compliance with each individual data element, clinicians can determine the stability of the critical pathway process and initiate the identification of process issues.

Descriptive Analysis: Run Chart

◆ Timing of Physical Therapy Initiation

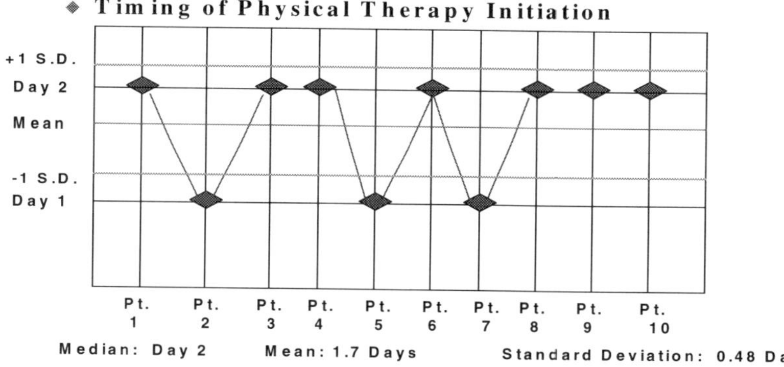

Median: Day 2 Mean: 1.7 Days Standard Deviation: 0.48 Days

Individual critical pathway elements can be analyzed to determine where deviations occur most frequently along the pathway. Determining where variances occur in the pathway helps focus investigation on reasons for the variance.

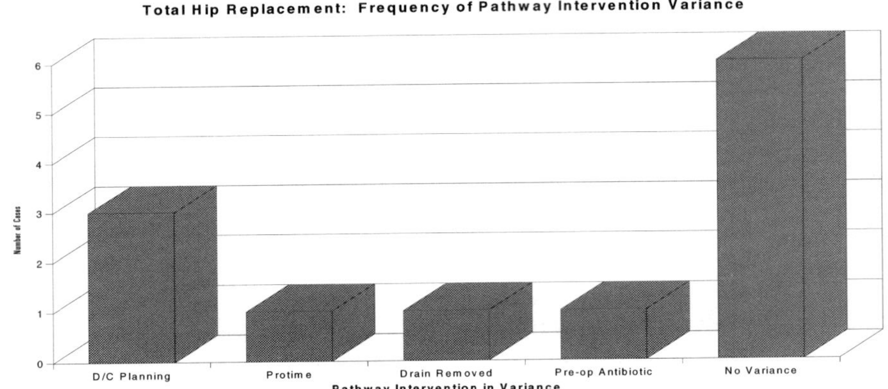

Analyzing critical pathway elements can help practitioners to determine the presence or absence of deviations. However, this analysis does not explain why deviations occur or how deviations affect the outcome of the case. To understand either of these aspects, clinicians need to incorporate information about variation issues and outcome data.

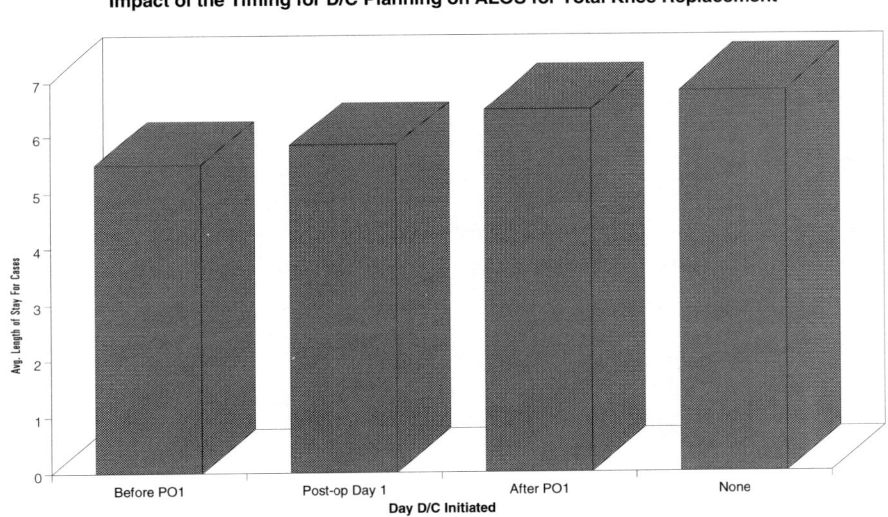

Clinicians' Performance

A second type of pathway analysis compares individual caregiver practices with the aggregated practice of the group. This comparison can be accomplished by distributing aggregated data to practitioners along with their own performance data.

Practitioner Peer Comparison

Critical Pathway Element: Congestive Heart Failure	Aggregated Results for January through March		Your Results for January through March	
	# of Cases	% of Cases	# of Cases	% of Cases
Assessed dyspnea level daily	40/50	80%	2/10	20%
Ordered diuretics	50/50	100%	10/10	100%
Ordered ACE inhibitor	20/50	40%	5/10	50%
Ordered oxygen only when pulse oximetry reading below 94%	20/20	100%	5/5	100%
Ordered oxygen when pulse oximetry above 94%	10/20	50%	0/5	0%
Patient Outcomes:	# of Cases	Avg.	# of Cases	Avg.
LOS	50	6.8	10	4.8
Respiratory Failure	50	6%	10	0%
Readmission w/i 30 days	50	4%	10	10%

Reasons for Variance

Once a deviation from a critical pathway is found, the reason for this variance needs to be investigated by the case manager in collaboration with the care manager and caregivers. The reasons for variances are then aggregated and analyzed to:

- Identify opportunities for improvements
- Assist with targeting future pathway populations

Clinicians can develop a sequence of pareto charts to help identify the major reasons for variations in data. The resulting analysis can serve as a springboard for continuous quality improvement teams, future education programs, revision of the pathway or the development of a new pathway.

By counting the number of times a deviation occurs for a particular reason, clinicians can focus their efforts on eliminating the cause of the deviation. For example:

> Clinicians in Hospital Anywhere notice that 40 percent of the time surgery for the repair of a fractured hip is performed on Day 2 instead of Day 1. When this deviation is explored further, it is discovered the reason for the sixteen (16) delays were for five (5) main reasons: eight (8) were for operative suites not available, four (4) were for patient conditions, two (2) were for no anesthesiologist available, one (1) was for no orthopaedic surgeon available, and one (1) because the patient delayed treatment. This information can be displayed in a pareto chart to highlight the area which has the biggest impact on improving compliance with a critical pathway.

By focusing on the few reasons that will change 60-80 percent of the outcomes, clinicians can improve patient care more effectively.

Pareto Chart

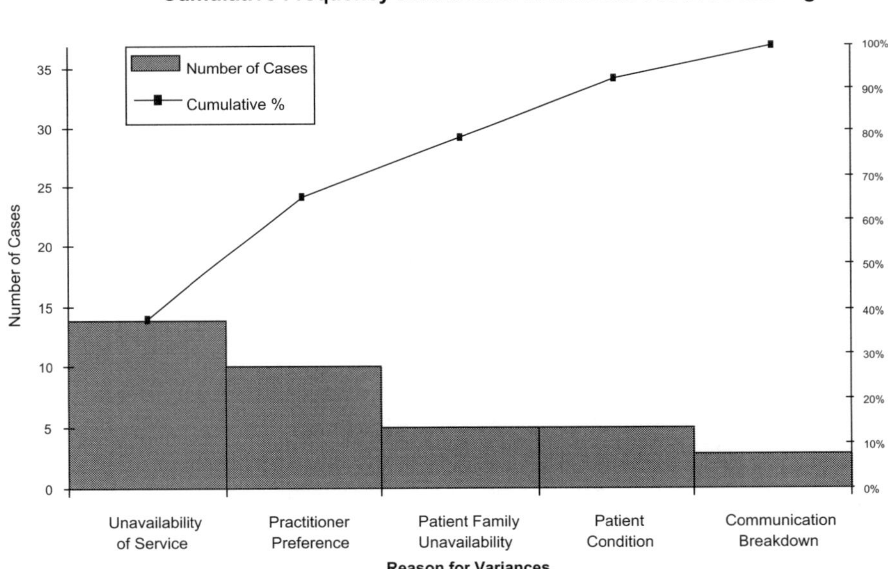

Patient Outcomes

The final type of analysis concerns outcome measurements, which evaluate:

- The attainment of established pathway goals
- Comparisons between cases that complied with, to cases which deviated from, the pathway

- Correlations between critical pathway elements and patient outcomes

In addition to these three main outcome analyses, clinicians may wish to compare outcomes to those found in outside data sources.

Established pathway goals can serve as benchmarks for evaluating actual critical pathway outcomes. By making this analysis, clinicians can determine if the implemented pathway actually improves care or if modifications to the pathway need to be considered so the established goals can be met.

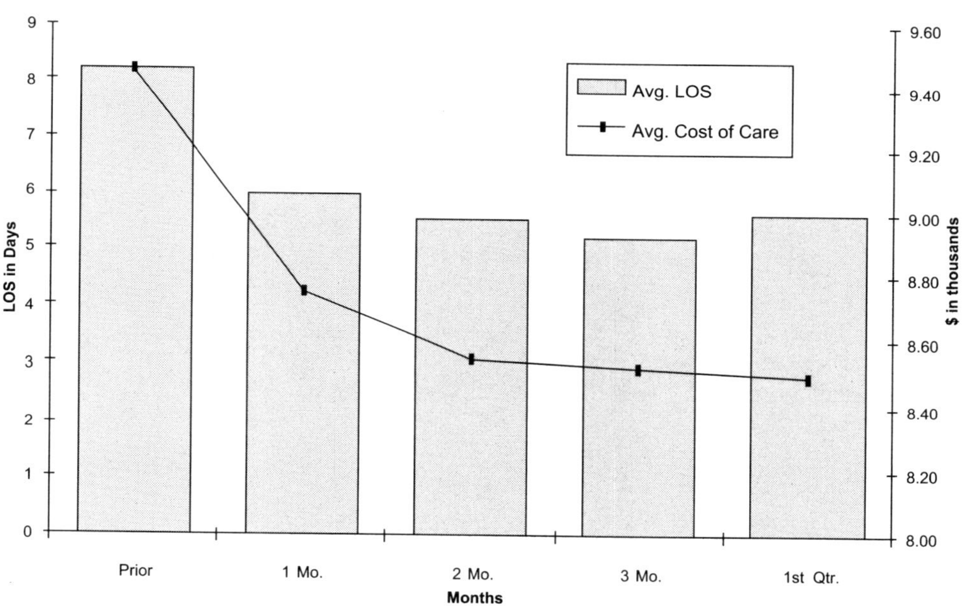

To determine if the established critical pathway process is the most effective method to deliver patient care, comparisons must be made between cases which follow the pathway and those which deviate.

Pathway Elements: Analysis

- **Validate Original Decisions**
  - **Correlation coefficient: 0.35 (Fair degree of relationship)**
  - **Chi square test: 8.948 (Significant 0.10)**

			Time Period for Data									
			Prior to Path		Mo 1		Mo 2		Mo 3		Group Summary	
			# of Cases	ALOS	# of Cases	ALOS	# of Cases	ALOS	# of Cases	ALOS	# of Cases	ALOS
Pathway Elements Which Impact ALOS	D/C Planning	According to Path	13	5.8	10	5	9	5.1	6	4.83	38	5.29
		Earlier than Path	3	5.5	2	5	2	5	4	4.5	11	4.9
		Later than Path	22	6.5	3	6.3	3	7	1	6	29	6.52
		None	6	6.8	1	8	0				7	7
		Total	44	6.4	16	5.4	14	5.5	11	4.8	85	

- **Revise Pathway Elements Using Data**
  - **Reflect changes in practice**
  - **Refine timing, duration, and interventions**
  - **Link changes to desired outcomes**

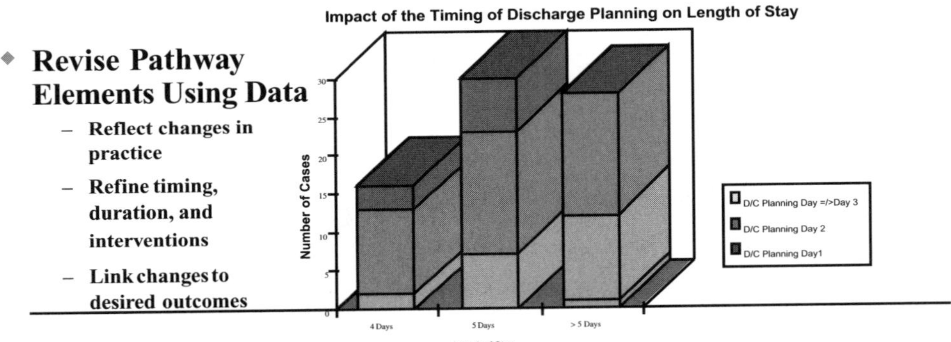

The final outcome analysis relates to correlating pathway processes to established outcomes. By correlating each pathway data element to actual outcomes, clinicians can determine the validity of their original conclusions.

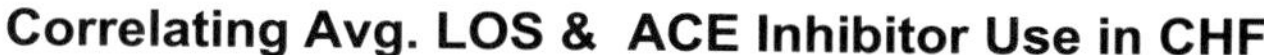

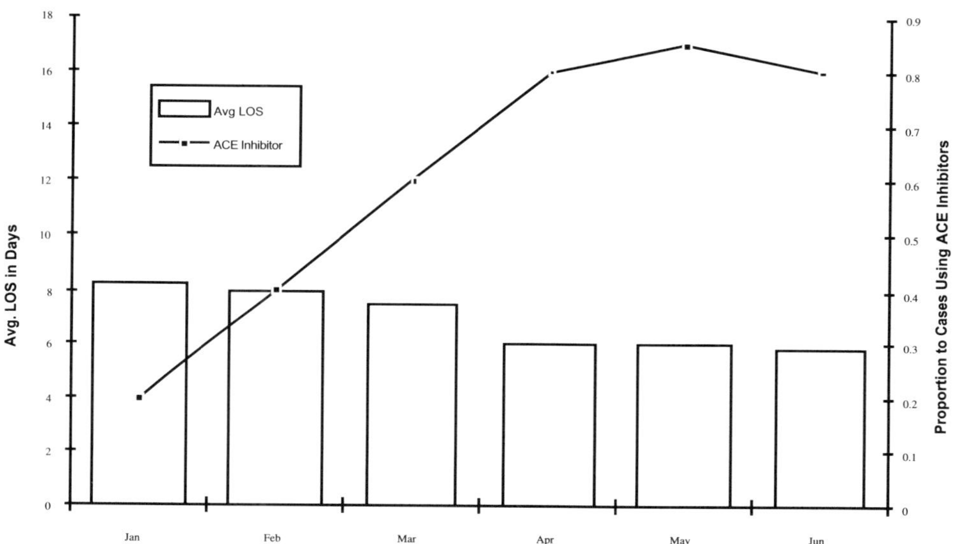

By collecting and analyzing data on pathway elements, reasons for variance and outcome measurements, clinicians can discover ways to improve patient care through staff education, process changes and system improvement.

4

Utilization of Critical Pathway Results

Introduction

The final step in the QTA Five Step Critical Pathway Process, utilization of pathway results, focuses on managing critical pathways through a changing health care environment, population shifts and the emergence of new technologies and practice guidelines. By effectively using pathway results, clinicians can sustain the improvements realized during pathway implementation, demonstrate the accomplishment of stated goals and foster "buy-in" for future critical pathway projects.

To accomplish this, methods need to be developed to:

- Reinforce desired performance
- Identify triggers for revising and updating pathways
- Implement critical pathway revisions

Reinforcement of Desired Performance

Clinicians can promote pathway compliance and remove impediments to desired results by effectively using the critical pathway data previously collected and analyzed. Attainment of desired results can be encouraged by providing positive reinforcement and relevant feedback to practitioners and eliminating pathway impediments.

While desired performance is positively reinforced, persistent non-compliance by practitioners may lead to counseling and/or sanctions in accordance with organizational policy.

Promoting Pathways through Positive Reinforcement

A consistent positive reinforcement system increases the probability that desired behaviors will become the new "standards of practice." To successfully implement a positive reinforcement system, clinicians need to follow these specific principles:

- Reinforce specific behaviors
- Reward achievements as soon as possible
- Administer rewards consistently and impartially
- Reinforce all desired behaviors not just changes to desired behaviors
- Provide a variety of rewards

One of the simplest and most effective mechanisms for reinforcing critical pathways is to communicate positive results to clinicians, administrators and groups within the organization and to appropriate outside agencies. Communication about critical pathway performance and outcomes can be accomplished through verbal announcements, presentation of pathway results or written acknowledgments of contributions.

Besides acknowledging positive results of pathways, some organizations have developed monetary reward systems for desired pathway compliance and attainment of goals.

It is especially important to understand the precedent established by a financial reward system and to take measures to clearly communicate the reasons for the reward.

Promoting Desired Pathway Results through Feedback

Feedback of pathway results informs clinicians about how they are meeting established expectations and assists them in planning future pathway related activities. Based on their awareness of pathway results, individual clinicians can adjust their practice, compare their performance to group norms and initiate education to improve their knowledge, skills and abilities.

Information about areas of compliance, areas of deviations and the reasons for deviations can assist clinicians in performing self-assessment. Practitioner information needs to be specific, accurate and delivered in a non-judgmental manner to protect self-esteem.

Sharing information regarding group performance and the attainment of pathway goals allows clinicians to identify pathway revisions, plan future pathways and make recommendations for continuous quality improvement (CQI) team activities.

One important issue regarding the sharing of practitioner information is the maintenance of confidentiality. This confidentiality is essential to remain in compliance with the peer review act in most states.

Promoting Pathway Compliance through Removal of Impediments

The final area for reinforcing desired performance deals with the removal of impediments to critical pathways. These impediments can include:

- Non-supportive policies and procedures
- Absence of necessary equipment, space, services or staff
- Insufficient knowledge, skills or abilities to perform the required actions

By using critical pathway variance data, clinicians can spot the major causes for pathway variances and take measures to eliminate them.

Once an impediment has been identified, clinicians can make referrals to appropriate individuals or groups. Each referral should be accompanied by the reason for the request and the supporting data so the improvement process can be initiated with a clear understanding of what needs to be changed and why.

When an impediment relates to insufficient knowledge, a request for specific continuing education programs or in-services can be sent to the organization's education department. When a system variance relating to delays in getting laboratory results is identified, a request for a laboratory focus team can be submitted to the CQI Steering Committee. By identifying and referring non-clinical issues, critical pathways integrate with the organization's existing CQI philosophy and efforts.

Identification of Triggers

Triggers are conditions or events that precipitate an evaluation and/or revision of the current critical pathway. For an event to qualify as a trigger, it must have a sustained impact on the health care environment. Special events are not triggers.

The three main categories of pathway triggers are:

- Practitioner
- Institutional
- Community

Practitioner Triggers

Practitioner triggers include events or conditions that alter practitioners' compliance with established pathways. These triggers generally deal with changes in established practice guidelines, new technologies and treatment modalities or changes in available clinical expertise. Pathway data reflects these changes as:

- Low or decreasing compliance rates for specific critical pathway elements
- Unmet pathway goals
- Superior outcomes for practitioners not in compliance with pathways
- Increased deviations from the pathway due to practitioner issues

Each organization needs to establish its own control limits for trigger related data. Control limits are the boundaries of acceptable variation within the critical pathway process. When a control limit is exceeded, clinicians need to evaluate the reasons for the variance to determine if a pathway revision should be initiated.

Institutional Triggers

Institution based triggers are the conditions or events occurring within an organization that impact the services available to customers. These triggers include additions, eliminations or revisions to the organization's services, programs or technologies.

Common institutional triggers include:

- Revision in the vision or mission statement for the organization

- Purchase or initiation of a new alternate level of care, such as a rehabilitation facility, home health services or ambulatory surgical center
- Purchase of new equipment
- Development or discontinuation of a patient care service within an organization

These triggers may be identified by an increase in system variances or by a request from clinicians to revise the current pathway boundaries or elements.

Community Triggers

Community based triggers relate to the conditions or events that impact the population served by a health care organization. When a change in the community occurs, the organization needs to consider revising existing critical pathways or initiating new critical pathways.

Community based factors may require critical pathway revisions if any of the following conditions are present:

- A steadily increasing number of patient variances
- Changes in the demographic profile of clients
- Changes in the types of reimbursement
- An increase in patient complaints about the care provided

Implementing Pathway Revisions

Critical pathway revision requires a systematic mechanism incorporating many of the same activities found in the development and implementation steps in the overall critical pathway process. The revision process integrates these activities with an organization's CQI process.

Who Can Initiate a Revision?

Because critical pathways are a multi-disciplinary process, anyone should be able to initiate a change in an existing pathway or propose a new one. By allowing multiple points of initiation, joint responsibility and a team concept are reinforced, while proprietary interests are discouraged.

TABLE 7. The revision process integrates with the organization's CQI process.

Critical Pathway Steps	Pathway Components	CQI Steps
1. Identification of Target Population and Pathway Boundaries	• Develop selection criteria • Review available data • Select a patient population • Define pathway boundaries • Select pathway development groups	**F**ind a process to Improve **O**rganize a team
2. Development of Critical Pathway	• Establish critical pathway goals • Review literature and research • Hypothesize "how to" meet goals • Collect internal practice data • Analyze data for relationships to outcomes • Formulate pathway • Ratify resulting clinical process/ pathway	**C**larify current knowledge of the process **U**nderstand sources of process variations **S**elect the process improvement

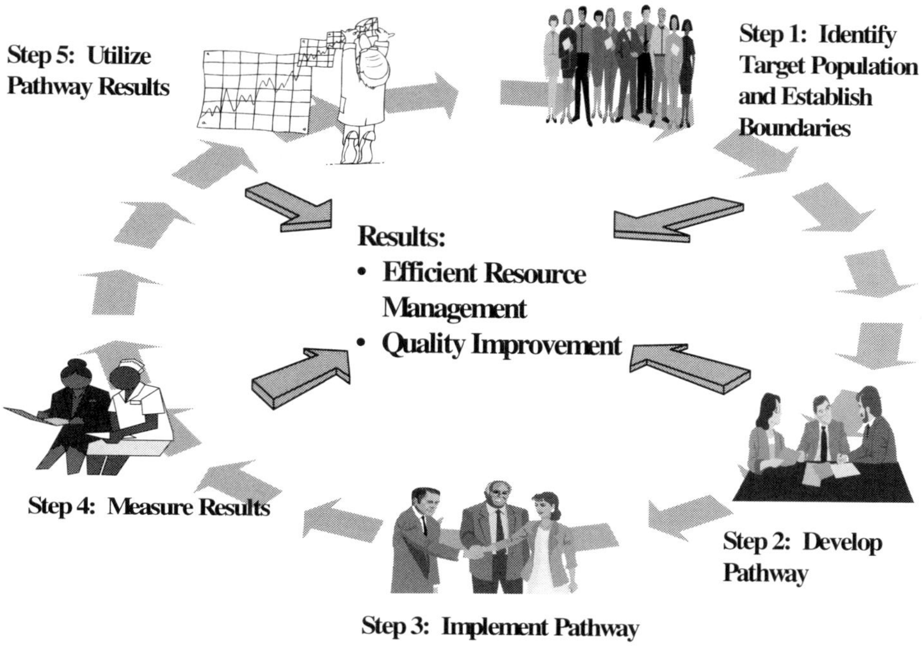

Step 1: Identify Target Population and Establish Boundaries

Step 2: Develop Pathway

Step 3: Implement Pathway

Step 4: Measure Results

Step 5: Utilize Pathway Results

Results:
- Efficient Resource Management
- Quality Improvement

5

Determining Fiscal Impact of Improved Clinical Processes

Introduction

With increased awareness of health care costs and emphasis on "value added activities," quality management professionals need to be able to analyze available financial information. This skill will allow them to:

- Determine the financial health of an organization
- Demonstrate the cost-benefit of quality initiative
- Determine the financial impact of future clinical improvements

Determining Financial Health

One of the skills required of all managers in health care is a basic understanding of financial reports, such as cash flow statements, balance sheets and income statements.

Financial Statements Present the Health of an Organization

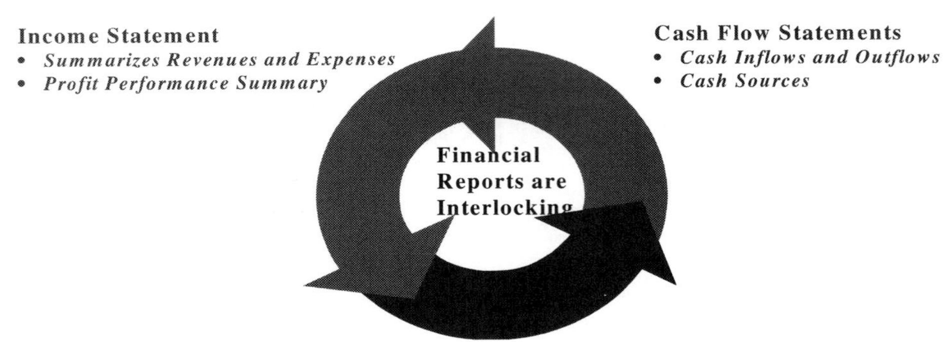

Cash flow statements provide information about the movement of cash, revenue sources and availability of cash. The income statement, also called a profit and loss statement, provides information about the profitability of an organization. The balance sheet presents a snapshot of the organizations financial condition at a given moment in time. The balance sheet lists all assets, including cash, accounts receivable, inventory, prepaid expenses, property, plant and equipment minus depreciation and all liabilities and equity.

Why is it important for quality professionals to know about financial statements? Simply put, quality and resources impact the bottom line of health care organizations. For example, if an organization receives most of its revenue from indemnity insurance plans, then reducing the length of stay could negatively impact the bottom line of the organization.

Income Statements Can Reflect Impact of Quality/Resource Initiatives

Fee-for-Service Charges Correlate with LOS Reductions

Fixed Charges are Unaffected with LOS Reductions

Hospital Anywhere: Income Statement		**Hospital Anywhere: Income Statement**	
Income Statement for One Month Ending 1/31/97		Income Statement for One Month Ending 1/31/97 Adjusted for Length of Stay/Reduction	
Service Revenues		Service Revenues	
Medicare	$1,400,000	Medicare	$1,400,000
Medicaid	$750,000	Medicaid	$750,000
Private Insurance	$2,280,000	Private Insurance	$2,052,000
HVD	$500,000	HVD	$500,000
Capitated	$750,000	Capitated	$750,000
Self	$10,000	Self	$9,000
Gross Margin	**$5,690,000**	**Gross Margin**	**$5,461,000**
Operating Expenses		**Operating Expenses**	
Wages	$2,560,500	Wages	$2,560,500
Workers Comp & Taxes	$614,520	Workers Comp & Taxes	$614,520
Benefits	$512,100	Benefits	$612,100
Supplies Expenses	$1,422,500	Supplies Expenses	$1,365,250
Insurance	$10,000	Insurance	$10,000
Contract Labor	$0	Contract Labor	$0
Depreciation Expense	$112,000	Depreciation Expense	$112,000
Mortage	$10,000	Mortgage	$10,000
Utilities	$3,500	Utilities	$3,500
Interest Expenses	$850	Interest Expenses	$850
Total Operating Expenses	**$5,245,970**	**Total Operating Expenses**	**$5,188,720**
Net Margin Before Taxes	$444,030	Net Margin Before Taxes	$272,280
Income Taxes	$66,605	Income Taxes	$40,842
NET MARGIN	**$377,426**	**NET MARGIN**	**$231,438**

By being aware of how the income statement is computed and the organization's case mix, clinicians and managers can target quality and resource activities at areas which will be mutually beneficial for patients and the organization.

Proving the Cost Benefit of Quality Initiatives

With growing emphasis on cost-containment and increasing pressure to prove "value added," many quality initiatives may be questioned in the future by administration and consumers regarding the benefits of making changes. Clinicians will need to answer these questions with both qualitative and quantitative data.

Some of the main reasons for analyzing the financial costs and benefits of quality initiatives include:

- Determining if a quality initiative is cost-effective

- Identifying tangible benefits
- Determining return on investment

To determine the cost benefit of a particular quality or resource initiative, the net financial benefit needs to be calculated. This calculation consists of the difference between the financial benefits and the financial costs contributed to produce the improvement result.

Financial Benefits - Costs = Cost Benefit (Net Benefit)

To start this computation process, there needs to be a review of the organizational goals for quality initiatives. The organizational goal is the outcome measurement for supporting the quality initiative and will answer the question "Why should I support this effort?" Organizational goals are not limited to only patient outcomes or financial contributions but will include employee and market benefits.

Organizational Goals Gives Clues For Determining Cost-Benefits

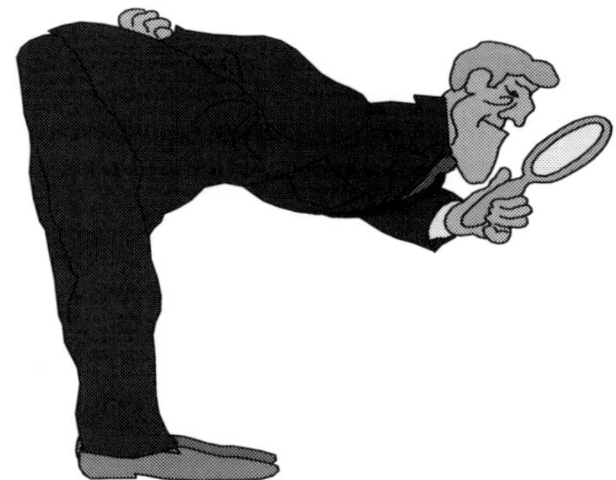

- ◆ **Improved patient outcomes**
- ◆ **Improved service**
- ◆ **Improved customer satisfaction**
- ◆ **Improved cost effectiveness**
- ◆ **Improved working environment**
- ◆ **Improved competitive position**

Once goals are selected for the quality initiative, the scope of costs and benefits included in the analysis should be determined. It is best to focus on short-term financial impact because these impacts are the easiest to defend and they demonstrate a correlation with the quality improvement.

Exclude Long-Run Benefits in Cost Benefit Analysis: Too Many Variables

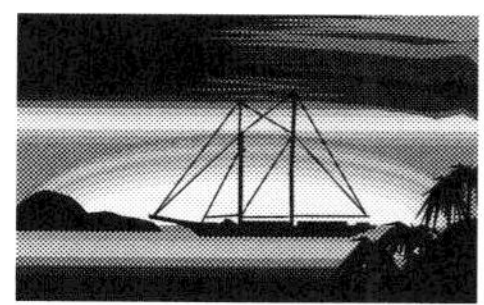

Non-financial impacts
- ***Better work environment***

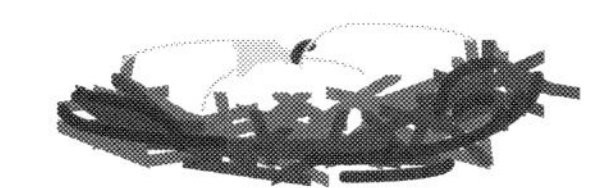

Financial benefits of satisfied customers
- ***Don't count your chickens before they hatch***

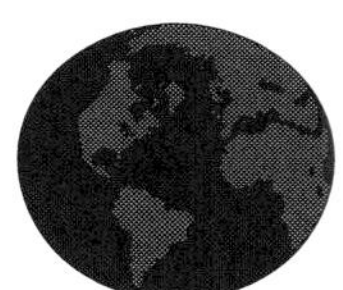

Benefits and costs of changes made outside formal improvement initiative

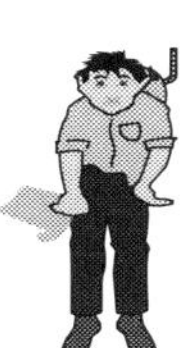

Reduced staff turnover, training costs, and labor grievances
- ***Employee issues dependent on multiple factors***

Adjustments for price/cost changes, except present time
- ***Can't predict the future***

The guidelines for calculating cost benefits include:

- Select how cost and benefits will be measured. The two most common options are:
  - Measuring all costs and benefits
  - Using only marginal costs and benefits
- Define financial terms used in the analysis
- Specify specific inclusions and exclusions from calculations
- Determine the number of years for calculating the cost benefits
- Select a starting date for calculations

- Use present value of all centralized and project costs and benefits if initiatives cover multiple years

TABLE 8.

Terminology	Definition	Example
Financial Costs	Net marginal costs plus net revenue losses.	Reallocation of staff without experiencing an increase in payroll costs is $0.00 financial costs.
Financial Benefits	Net marginal cost savings plus net revenue increases.	If the cost of care for patients with bacterial pneumonia is decreased by $500.00 and the profit margin is increased by $200.00 then the financial benefit is $700.00 a patient.
Capital Cost Impact	Use depreciation rate as annual cost of all capital expenditures directly related to improvement.	A new computer system is purchased, depreciation is used as the capital cost impact.
Implementation Cost Impact	Length of training time X (Number of employees, physicians, etc. X cost of employees time) Only additional time worked will be included.	The cost for training 200 staff nurses for 1 hour on the use of a congestive heart failure pathway resulted in 60 staff had 30 minutes of overtime. 60 X 0.5 X $37.50= $1125.00
One-time Benefits and Costs	One time benefits and costs need to be computed for the first year benefits and costs.	A construction project is canceled because of a reduction in the emergency department waiting time makes the construction unnecessary.
Centralized Costs	Consultants, training materials, facilities and equipment, supplies, and promotion or celebration costs.	An outside consultant on how to develop critical pathways.
Centralized Benefits	Income received from speaking and consulting fees and sale of materials developed.	After developing an automated nursing documentation system for home care, the system was marketed to other agencies.

Once the decision rules are determined, it is time to estimate the financial costs and benefits of a quality or resource initiative. An example of a cost benefit analysis is shown below.

Cost Benefit Analysis of a Pneumonia Critical Pathway

- **Organizational Goals**
  - **Reduce the average length of stay from 6 days to 4 days.**
  - **Improve reimbursement**
  - **Reduce transfers to ICU**
- **Scope of Costs and Benefits (Marginal)**

Costs of Pathway	Benefits of Pathway
• Overtime for team meetings • Overtime for implementation training • Outside printing costs • Added staff for case management • Cost of food at meetings	• Reduction in the patient care costs • Increase in revenues • Sale of completed pathway

Pneumonia Benefit Analysis

- **Bacteria Pneumonia**
  - **165 Cases a year**
  - **Average cost of case: $4000.00**
  - **Average reimbursement per case: ($500.00)**
  - **Total profit/loss: ($82,500.00)**
- **New Pathway**
  - **165 Cases a year**
  - **Average cost per case: $3300.00**
  - **Average reimbursement per case: $200.00**
  - **Total profit/loss: $33,000.00**
- **Financial Benefits**
  - **Reduction or increase in cost: $ 700.00 per case**

Pneumonia Cost Analysis

- **Marginal Cost of Developing Pathway**
  - Overtime for Staff: $0.00
  - Overtime for Implementation Training: $500.00
  - New Equipment: $0.00
  - Printing Cost of Forms: $5000.00
  - Food Costs: $300.00
- **Project Costs:** $5,800.00
- **Cost Benefit of Quality Initiative**
  - » $231,000.00 - $5,800.00 = $225,200

After the cost analysis is completed, a report highlighting all benefits, both tangible and intangible, needs to be written and submitted for review. The financial benefits and costs need to be reviewed by financial analysts and managers to obtain concurrence with the results.

Communicate, Communicate, Communicate

- **Communicate widely so costs, benefits and returns are well understood**
- **Use multiple communication methods**

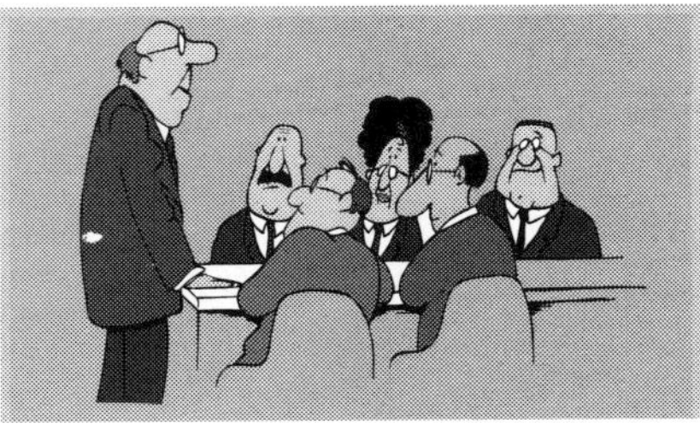

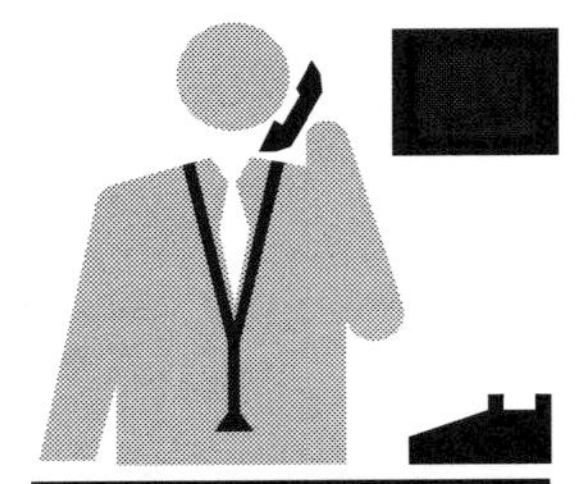

6

Relationship between Critical Pathways and Case Management

Introduction

One of the recent solutions proposed by the health care industry for managing clinical quality and resources is the concept of case management. The goal of case management is to coordinate and manage the delivery of patient care services throughout the continuum of care. Because case management is evolutionary, there is frequent confusion about a number of issues:

- What is case management?
- What is the difference between case management and critical pathways?
- Can an organization use critical pathways without having a case management program?
- Can an organization have case management without pathways?

To start answering these questions and others, a generic definition for case management needs to be established. The case management definition that will be used in the following discussion is:

> Case management is a collaborative effort that coordinates the delivery of essential services to customers within in the health care system.

The current application of case management in health care organizations is through individuals, the case managers, who focus on managing a single case during an episode of care. There are several core principles which form the basis for case management. These principles include:

- The principle of empowered customer representative. For case management to be successful, the individual assigned to this role needs to have the authority to make decisions and initiate actions in behalf of the patient.

- The principle of collaboration. Case management is not a person or a team but a process which facilitates collaboration and coordination among all providers of care.

- The principle of flexibility. Because patients require different amounts and types of services based on their clinical conditions, environment, social support and economic situation, case management needs to be flexible enough to meet these needs.

- The principle of "good care is cost effective care." One of the basic beliefs of case management advocates is that by providing coordinated consistent care to customers quality will improve and costs will be reduced. The basis for this belief is that costs can be reduced without sacrificing quality and safety through the reduction of duplications, delays and oversights.

- The principle of probability. **One of the basic tools of case management is the critical/clinical pathway.** This tool is based on the analysis of aggregated practice and outcome data. By using a pathway, cases managers are really applying a plan of care which has the greatest probability of meeting the average patient's needs.

Current Case Management Models

Currently, there are five principal case management models used in the health care system. The basic intent and required expertise for each model varies based on the environment in which case management functions are performed. The models are:

- **Self-care model**: This is a health promotion model which casts the customer as the case manager. This educational model focuses on preventing illness and promoting health. Because patients are responsible for coordinating their own care, the health care team serves only as consultants.

- **Primary care model**: This model uses the primary care provider, generally a physician or nurse practitioner, as the case manager or gatekeeper. This model encompasses many episodes of care and crosses different levels of care. The intent of this model is to provide consistent and coordinated care to a single patient. The secondary intent is to control clinical costs by serving as a gatekeeper for referrals.
- **Episodic care model**: The episodic care model is currently the most frequently found case management model today. This model is generally facility or organizationally based and focuses on providing efficient, cost effective care. Currently, nurses are the predominant case managers for this model.
- **Social service model**: The social service model is probably the oldest type of case management found. This model focuses on providing the environmental, financial and emotional support required by a customer to optimize independence and safety. Generally, this model appears in social service agencies and people with social work background serve as the case managers.
- **Catastrophic care model**: Usually, when a patient experiences a catastrophic illness or injury, their third-party payer assigns a case manager to coordinate and manage all patient services related to that condition. The intent of this model is to control costs by finding the most economical means for providing care. Case management services are provided across the continuum of care as they relate to the catastrophic condition. These case management services are provided by either the third party payer or brokered to an independent case management company.

Common case management characteristics can be discovered by reviewing the current models. These characteristics are present regardless of who is performing case management or where the function is located within the health care system. These common characteristics are:

- Case management is patient focused
- It involves coordination of services provided to a patient
- It is by nature collaborative, with multiple practitioner involvement
- Motivation for case management is either resource or quality management

There are several characteristics, missing in the current case management models, which need to be present to meet the changing needs of the health care system. These missing ingredients for successful case management are:

- Holistic approach to patients' health, instead of episodic attention to illness. By converting the focus of case management from disease control to wellness promotion, longitudinal benefits can be realized.
- A systems approach to case management which is based on aggregated clinical and financial data analysis instead of anecdotal case management notes.

By combining the strengths from each of the existing case management models with the additional characteristics noted above, a new **Health Coordination Model** emerges. This model focuses on providing coordinated health care services throughout a patient's life. The goal is to optimize a person's health through preventative efforts and coordinated care, thus producing long-term savings instead of short-term gains.

As capitated programs expand and information management technologies develop, this model will become feasible. Also, case management programs will move from being strictly institution-based to health-network-based, supporting a truly coordinated health care system.

A suggested composition of a case management team is a care manager with the clinical expertise to collaborate in clinical care coordination, a case manager, with the expertise to manage the financial aspects of the patient and an information specialist who can supply the process, outcome and financial data required for continued improvement. Each case team would support several physicians and nurse practitioners, who still retain the primary responsibility for patient care.

Relationship between Case Management and Critical Pathways

Frequently people are confused about the difference between case management and critical pathways and will use the terms interchangeably.

Critical pathways, clinical pathways, protocols and the like are the standardized plans of care being delivered to patients. Pathways define a process with a beginning and an end. This process may include only one level of care or may cross the continuum of care. Organizations can have critical pathways without having a case management program.

Case management is a means for managing care and is a composite discipline. Because case managers do not have the authority or expertise to independently decide how to care for a patient, they need a set of standardized tools.

These tools can be critical pathways, clinical pathways or protocols. Case management, as it is used currently, cannot exist without pre-established plans of care.

Appendix A

Sample Pathway Policy and Procedure

Many organizations use policies and procedures to standardize, formalize and communicate processes. These policies also serve as a reference for staff decisions and actions. Because of such wide scale use of policies and procedures, we have included an example of a critical pathway policy and procedure.

However, this is just one example of how an institution could standardize the critical pathway process and communicate pathway guidelines and procedures. There is no universal policy that fits all organizations. Policies should reflect an organization's infrastructure and be consistent with actual practice in order to be relevant and useful.

CRITICAL PATHWAY PROCESS

Health Care Organization Anywhere

I. **PURPOSE:** To state policy, define terminology, assign responsibilities and outline procedures for the development, implementation and maintenance of critical pathways.

II. **POLICY:** It is the policy of this health care organization that critical pathways will be used to promote consistent, cost-effective and high quality care.

III. **DEFINITIONS:**

a. **Critical Pathways:** Clinical guidelines for the timing and provision of care. These guidelines will include only the care elements proven to support desired patient care outcomes and agreed to by involved caregivers. For a guideline to be considered a critical pathway, it must be endorsed by the Critical Pathway Steering Committee and ratified by the Medical Executive Committee.

b. **Variances:** All deviations from the pathway schedule of clinical assessments or interventions.

c. **Patient Variance:** A deviation from the critical pathway caused by a change in a patient's condition, unavailability or actions.

d. **System Variance:** A deviation from the critical pathway caused by breakdown or unavailability of either services, supplies, medications or equipment.

e. **Practitioner Variance:** A deviation from the critical pathway caused by an omission or commission by a caregiver without evidence of a system or patient variance.

IV. **RESPONSIBILITIES.**

a. *The President* is responsible for providing leadership and administrative support for the critical pathway development and implementation process.

b. *The Critical Pathway Steering Committee* is responsible for facilitating and endorsing the development and implementation of critical pathways. The committee will establish critical pathway process policies and procedures, sanction pathway activities, endorse completed pathways and develop infrastructure required for pathway maintenance, communication, education and evaluation.

c. *Medical Executive Committee* is responsible for recommending areas for critical pathway development, reviewing and ratifying all pathways, and taking actions to encourage pathway compliance. These actions include, but are not limited to, planning continuing medical education programs, assigning members to development teams and supporting peer review activities.

d. *The Critical Pathway Coordinator* is responsible for coordinating the critical pathway process under the direction of the Critical Pathway Steering Committee. This position coordinates and facilitates critical pathway development and implementation by providing administrative and technical support to critical pathway teams, care managers and caregivers. The coordinator will collaborate with involved clinicians to prepare, present and analyze critical pathway data. This position serves as a critical pathway consultant and educator within the organization.

e. *All Vice Presidents* are responsible for facilitating the participation by services under their supervision in support of critical pathway development and implementation processes.

f. *Clinical Service Directors* are responsible for supporting critical pathways through the identification of potential pathways, assignment of staff to specific teams and communication and reinforcement of desired pathway outcomes.

g. *Care Managers* are responsible for collaborating with other treatment team members to facilitate appropriate pathway compliance, managing appropriate application of pathways, coordinating care within a health care organization and documenting patient care.

h. *Case Managers* are responsible for monitoring application of pathways, investigating the reason for variances, facilitating continuity of care within the health care system and documenting variances and corrective actions taken to facilitate pathway compliance.

i. *The Attending Physician* is responsible for initiating and discontinuing a critical pathway. The attending physician will serve as the manager for all medical care provided to the patient. If a variance is noted in the medical care, the attending physician is responsible for either correcting the variance or documenting why it occurred.

j. *The Nursing Education Department* is responsible for providing orientation to critical pathways and coordination of continuing and in-service education programs related to critical pathway knowledge, skills and abilities.

k. *Critical Pathway Development Team Members* are responsible for participating in critical pathway development and implementation through the timely completion of assignments, attendance at scheduled meetings, communication to peers, analysis of data and provision of education.

l. *Caregivers* are responsible for recommending potential critical pathways, providing input into pathway development and revisions, utilizing critical pathways and documenting patient care and variances according to established medical records procedures.

V. PROCEDURES.

a. Pathway Development and Implementation:

1. Critical pathways will be developed using a multi-disciplinary approach.
2. Every critical pathway development team will have at least one physician member or advisor.
3. Members of the development team are expected to attend 90 percent of the scheduled meetings.
4. Critical pathways will use the QTA methodology for developing and implementing critical pathways.
5. Progress reports on the team's efforts will be given a minimum of every two months to the involved departments and committees.
6. All critical pathways will be pilot tested prior to final endorsement and organization-wide implementation.

b. Utilization of a Pathway:

1. Critical pathways will be initiated by a physician order designating the appropriate critical pathway.
2. If an existing critical pathway is not ordered within four hours of admission or once a patient is diagnosed by a physician, then the patient's primary nurse will contact the attending physician. They will discuss the case to ascertain and document the reason for excluding the patient from the pathway. If the physician has already documented the reason for excluding the patient from the pathway in the medical record, the primary nurse will not contact the physician.
3. If a patient is admitted after 20:00 and the timeframes for the pathway are stated in days of care, then clinicians will record all care performed until midnight the following day (or for a maximum of 28 hours) in the area designated for Day One.

4. At the beginning of every workshift, a registered nurse will review the pathway and create a plan of care to accomplish the prescribed care and patient goals.

5. When a patient is transferred to another patient unit, the critical pathway will continue. The transferring nurse will inform the receiving nurse about the pathway and review the completed pathway elements.

6. When a patient on a pathway is discharged from one facility to another level of care, the pathway plan for aftercare will be documented on the discharge summary and reported to the receiving agency.

7. A patient can be removed from a critical pathway when the required care deviates significantly from the pathway. This decision must be made by two caregivers, one being the attending physician. To discontinue a pathway, the time, date and reason for discontinuation must be recorded in the medical record.

c. Pathway Documentation:

1. To initiate documentation of a critical pathway, obtain a copy of the appropriate critical pathway documentation form and stamp the form with the patient's addressograph card.

2. Record the current date and patient unit in the appropriate space.

3. When a critical element is performed, the person performing the assessment or intervention will initial on the space preceding the element. Assessments are recorded on the space following the relevant pathway element. If there is insufficient space, record assessments in the progress notes section of the form.

4. If a critical pathway element is not performed for any reason, leave the line preceding the pathway element blank. Record on the progress notes the reason for patient variances and record the actions taken to reinstate the pathway. If the variance is due to a system or practitioner issue, record only the actions taken to reinstate the pathway. System and practitioner variances will be recorded on the care management form.

5. Keep the current critical pathway medical record form and vital sign flow sheet in the patient's room or other appropriate place.

6. Record the date and time and sign your name (first initial, last name and title) on a line of the progress note section at the end of your shift. If, during your shift, you documented at least once in the progress notes, that will substitute for this step.

7. Place the critical pathway medical record forms in the progress notes section of the medical record when the patient is discharged or the pathway is discontinued.

8. Critical pathway documentation will conform to all medical records procedures.

9. To discontinue a pathway, record the date, time and the reason for discontinuation in the progress notes. Both caregivers making the decision should sign the progress note.

d. Case Management:

1. A case manager will be assigned to a patient within the first 24 hours of admission.

2. The case manager will monitor critical pathway compliance concurrently on a daily basis.

3. To begin the case management process, a case management plan will be obtained and the patient name, medical record number, prior approval number, admission date, insurance company and provisional diagnosis will be recorded in the appropriate spaces. The date of care will be placed in the appropriate heading for each timeframe for care. If a patient is admitted after 20:00, and the critical pathway is segmented into days of care, the "Day One" care will consist of all care provided until 24:00 on the following day.

4. If a clinical assessment or intervention was completed according to the pathway, the case manager will mark an X on the line preceding the critical pathway element.

5. If a clinical assessment or intervention did not occur as scheduled, the case manager will investigate the reason for the variance and take appropriate action to promote pathway compliance. To record these actions, the case manager will document the variance code on the line preceding the scheduled pathway element and record, in the case management action plan, the date of the variance, the appropriate variance and action codes, additional comments and initials.

6. If additional clinical actions (those not specified by the pathway) were performed, the care manager will record them in the critical pathway element cells that correspond to the designated time frame

and aspect of care. The reason for performing this action will be determined and placed on the line preceding the intervention. The case manager will then take appropriate actions and record, in the case management action plan section of the form the date of the variance, the appropriate variance and action codes, additional comments and his or her initials.

7. If a critical pathway element is not applicable, then the case manager will record code P1 on the line preceding the not applicable element and draw a line through the element.

8. Once the patient has been removed from the pathway, by either discontinuation of the pathway or patient discharge, the care manager will forward the completed form to the Critical Pathway Coordinator's office within 24 hours of discontinuation.

e. Pathway Revisions:

1. Revisions to established pathways can be initiated by any clinician or group of clinicians by submitting a completed opportunity statement to the Critical Pathway Steering Committee.

2. After the Critical Pathway Steering Committee sanctions the revision process a revision team will be appointed.

3. The revision process will follow the same procedures prescribed for pathway development.

f. Confidentiality: Confidentiality will exist for all care management records and documents created at this facility. This information may not be disclosed to any person or entity except in compliance with the Peer Review Act of this state. Identification of the individual patient and the caregivers will be withheld by appropriate means to assure confidentiality. Any requests for release of information pertaining to the facility's clinical quality improvement data must be cleared through the Director of Medical Records. Critical pathway documents will be maintained by the Critical Pathway Coordinator for a period of three years. These documents must be kept secure and confidential.

g. Conflict of Interest: Conflict of interest will be avoided by prohibiting a person from reviewing their own professional practice.

VI. REFERENCES: JCAHO-Accreditation Manual for Hospitals.

VII. RECISION: 9/1/96.

Appendix B

Glossary of Terms

AHCPR: Agency for Health Care Policy and Research.

Care Management Plan: A tentative course of action used to measure and manage patient care activities.

Care Manager: The individual assigned manage a specific patient's critical pathway activities. This term is synonymous with clinical case manager.

Case Manager: The individual assigned to measure and manage a specific patient's critical pathway activities, perform utilization review and coordinate discharge planning.

Clinical Pathway: Every element of care required on a daily basis throughout an episode of treatment, regardless of the impact on patient outcomes.

Critical Pathway Guide: A written copy of a critical pathway used to provide direction for clinical interventions and documentation of care. This guide can be a temporary or permanent part of the medical record.

Clinical Practice Guidelines: Statements which describe appropriate health care decisions and activities for a specific clinical condition. These statements can be developed by professional, regulatory, commercial or educational groups.

Clinician: Any individual who provides clinical care to patients. This term is used synonymously with caregiver and practitioner. For example, physicians, nurses and social workers are all practitioners.

Cluster Random Sample: A two stage sampling process which first sub-divides the population into groups or clusters according to a specific characteristic, then a random sample of clusters is chosen. A portion of subjects within each cluster are selected. This sampling method is most often used in epidemiological research and commonly based on geographic areas or districts.

Concurrent Review: The process of monitoring the care provided to patients during an episode of care. This term is synonymous with prospective review.

Consensus: A group decision that all members of the group accept and support.

CQI: Continuous Quality Improvement

Criteria: Standards or rules on which a judgment or decision can be based.

Critical Pathway: The few vital clinical activities in a treatment regimen proven to impact on the clinical or financial outcomes of care.

Decision Matrix: A decision support tool used to rank several options relative to a set of criteria.

Dependent Variable: An element in a study thats value is changed by the presence or absence of one or more other variables.

External Data Source: The point outside an organization where information originates.

External Triggers: Conditions or events outside the organization that precipitate an evaluation and/or revision of the current critical pathway.

Independent Variable: A factor in a study that is unchanged by the presence or absence of other variables.

Internal Data Source: The point within an organization where information is created.

Internal Triggers: Conditions or events within the organization that precipitate an evaluation and/or revision of the current critical pathway.

Matrix: An array of data shown in columns and rows.

Opportunity Statement: A concise statement to describe a process in need of improving, its boundaries, the reasons for concern and the expected benefits of improving the process.

Pathway Boundaries: The points of service where a pathway starts and where it ends.

Pathway Hypothesis: A statement describing a clinician's beliefs or educated guesses about the relationship between specific clinical elements and outcomes.

Patient Care Review Activities: The traditional clinical monitoring functions found in a health care organization. These functions include quality assurance and control, utilization review, risk management and infection control.

Patient Variance: A deviation from the critical pathway caused by a change in the patient's condition, or due to the availability, decisions or actions of the patient or his or her significant other.

Point of Service: A specific moment of time when a particular department or branch of a health care organization's staff provides specified patient care.

Practice Parameters: Elements of care promulgated by professional societies, regulatory agencies or published in literature which define the boundaries of safe clinical practice.

Practitioner: Any individual who provides clinical care to patients. This term is used synonymously with caregiver and clinician. Physicians, nurses and social workers (among others) are all practitioners.

Practitioner Variance: A deviation from the critical pathway caused by an omission or commission by a caregiver without evidence of a system or patient variance.

Pre-printed Physician Orders: Physician orders which are pre-printed but must be activated by a physician order.

QTA: Quality Team Associates.

Retrospective Review: The process of monitoring the care provided to patients after an episode of care is complete.

Scope of Pathway: The range of patient care services provided within the boundaries of a pathway.

Standards of Care: The level of assistance or treatment provided to those in need.

Standards of Practice: The level of performance demonstrated during the assistance or treatment of those in need.

Standing Orders: Diagnostic and treatment protocols which are activated without a physician order.

Simple Random Sample: A portion of items (cases) selected from a population in a manner which ensures all items have an equal chance or probability of being chosen.

Skill Assessment: An evaluation of the knowledge, skills and abilities required to perform a task.

Stratified Random Sample: Selecting a portion of a population by sub-dividing it according to specified characteristics, then randomly choosing cases from each sub-group.

Systematic Random Sample: A sampling method where every nth number of items is selected for the sample. "N" is a predetermined constant number of cases. For example, every seventh case will be included in the sample.

System Variance: A deviation from the critical pathway caused by breakdown or unavailability of services, information, supplies, medications or equipment.

Variance: Any deviation from the critical pathway schedule of clinical assessments and interventions regardless of its impact on patient outcomes.

Appendix C

Bibliography and References

Agency of Health Care Policy and Research. *Clinical Practice Guidelines*, U.S. Department of Health and Human Services, 1993.

American Academy of Orthopaedic Surgeons, "Femoral Neck Fracture (Adult)," *Clinical Policies*, Chicago. (Dec. 1990): 15-18.

Guidelines for Physiatric Practice and Inpatient Review Criteria. Board of Governance. Chicago: American Academy of Physical Medicine & Rehabilitation, Sept. 1989.

American Heritage Dictionary. 3d ed. (1992).

American Geriatrics Society (AGS) Position Statement CARE MANAGEMENT. AGS Board of Directors. New York, NY: American Geriatrics Society, April 1993.

Association for Practitioners in Infection Control. *The APIC Curriculum for Infection Control Practice*, 3 Vols. Dubuque: Kendall/Hunt, 1983. Vol. I.

Batalden, Paul and Buchanan, David. "Hospital Quality: Patient, Physician and Employee Judgments." *International Journal of Health Care Quality Assurance.* (Nov. 1990): 7-17.

Berwick, Donald M. "Sounding Board: Continuous Improvement as an Ideal in Health Care." *New England Journal of Medicine.* 320:1. (Jan.1989): 53-56.

Coile, Russel C. Jr. "Future Trends, Health Care Reform and the Outlook for Long-Term Care," *Journal of Long-Term Care Administration* (Fall 1993): 6-10.

Cribbin, James J. *Leader Skills for Executives.* Boston: Education for Management,1977.

Crosby, Philip B. *Quality Without Tears: The Art of Hassle-Free Management*, New York: McGraw-Hill, 1984.

Dawson-Saunders, Beth, and Trapp, Robert G. *Basic & Clinical Biostatistics*, Norwalk: Appleton & Lange, 1994.

Deming, W., Edwards. *Quality, Productivity, and Competitive Position*. Cambridge: M.I.T., 1982.

Donabedian, A.O. *Explorations in Quality Assessment and Monitoring. Vol. 1, The Definition of Quality and Approaches to Its Assessment*. Ann Arbor: Health Administration Press, 1980.

——. *Exploration in Quality Assessment and Monitoring. Vol.2, The criteria and Standards of Quality*. Ann Arbor: Health Administration Press, 1982.

——. *Exploration in Quality Assessment and Monitoring. Vol. 3, The Methods and Findings of Quality Assessment Monitoring: An Illustrated Analysis*. Ann Arbor: Health Administration Press, 1985.

Doyle, Richard L., *Healthcare Management Guidelines*, 5 Vols. San Francisco, CA: Milliman & Robertson, 1992. Vol. 2: Return-to-Work Planning.

Fanale, James E.; Keenan, Joseph M.; Hepburn, Kenneth W.; and Von Sternberg, Thomas. "Care Management," *Journal of American Geriatrics Society* 39:4, (April 1991): 431-437.

Gitlow, Howard S. And Shelly J. *The Deming Guide to Quality and Competitive Position*. Englewood Cliffs: Prentice-Hall, 1987.

Gronlund, Norman E. *Stating Objectives for Classroom Instruction*, 2d ed. New York: Macmillan, 1978.

Jader, Gary. "Ten Steps to Effective Persuasive Speaking," *Nursing Management* (March 1993): 46-48.

Joint Commission on Accreditation of Healthcare Organizations. 1994 Accreditation Manual for Hospitals Volume I. Chicago: 1993.

Joseph, Eric D. *Statistical Imperative*. Chicago: Care Education Group, 1993.

Juran, Joseph M. *Juran on Planning for Quality*. New York: The Free Press, 1988.

—— *Juran on Quality by Design: The New Steps for Planning Quality into Goods and Services*. New York: The Free Press, 1992.

—— *Juran's Quality Control Handbook*. New York: McGraw-Hill, 1988.

Kane, Robert L., Ouslander, Joseph G., and Itamar, Abrass B. *Essentials of Clinical Geriatrics*. 3d ed. New York: McGraw-Hill, 1994.

Kongstvedt, Peter R., *The Managed Health Care Handbook.* 2d ed. Gaithersburg, MD: Aspen Publication, 1993.

Leedy, Paul D., *Practical Research Planning and Design*, New York: Macmillan, 1980.

Lewis-Ford, Brenda Kay, "Management Techniques: Coping with Difficult People," *Nursing Management*, Vol. 24 (March 1993): 36-38.

McClelland, Eleanor; Kelly, Kathleen; and Kathleen C. Buckwalter, Continuity of Care: *Advancing the Concept of Discharge Planning*, Orlando: Grune & Stratton, 1985.

Shortell, Stephen M.; Morrison, Ellen M.; and Friedman, Bernard. *Strategic Choices for America's Hospitals*, San Francisco: Jossey-Bass, 1992.

Sloan, John P. *Protocols in Primary Care Geriatrics.* New York: Springer-Verlag, 1991.

Thompson, June M. et al., *Mosby's Clinical Nursing* 3d ed. St. Louis: Mosby, 1993.

Townsend, Patrick L. And Gebhardt, J.E. *Commit to Quality.* New York: Wiley, 1986.

VHA Tri-State Inc., *Continuous Quality Improvement: Strategies & Methods.* Nashville: Hospital Corporation of America, 1991.

Way, Lawrence W., *Current Surgical Diagnosis & Treatment.* 10 ed. Norwalk: Appleton & Lange, 1994.

Wall, Deborah K., and Joseph, Eric D. *Critical Pathways: Development and Implementation A Discussion Guide* Chicago: Care Communications, 1992.

———"Guidelines for Developing Critical Pathways" *Quality Management Update* 3:5 (May 1993): 6-8.

Wall, Deborah K., and Proyect, Mitchell M. *Moving From Parameters To Pathways: A Guide For Developing And Implementing Critical Pathways* Santa Cruz: Quality Team Associates, 1994.

———*Issues Which Impact Critical Pathway Success* Santa Cruz: Quality Team Associates, 1994.

White House Domestic Policy Council, The President's Health Security Plan, New York: Times Books, 1993.

Woolf, Steven H. "Practice Guidelines: A New Reality in Medicine III. Impact on Patient Care," *Archives of Internal Medicine.* 153 (Dec. 1993): 2646-2655.

Index

Acceptance, 21
ACE inhibitor use, 71
Application, inconsistent, 21
Attending physician, 23, 24, 99

Balance sheet, 84

Capital cost impact, 88
Caregiver, 100
Care manager, 48, 49, 99
Case for action, 12-13
Case coordinator, 24, 48
Case leader, 24
Case management
- action plan, 63
- application of, 91-92
- critical pathways relationship, 94-95
- guidelines, 102-3
- models, 92-93
- plan, 58-59
- plan, sample, 60-61

Case manager, 7, 47, 48, 49, 62, 99
Case team, 7
Case team members, 7
Case worker, 6-7
Cash flow statement, 84
Catastrophic care case management, 93
Centralization, 9-10
- of benefits, 88
- of costs, 88

Clinical pathway process, flow chart, 25
Clinical service directors, 99
Clinician performance, 67
Communication, 90
Community triggers, 77
Confidentiality, 103
Conflict of interest, 103
Congestive heart failure
- critical pathway peer comparison, 67
- systolic dysfunction, pathway, 30-32

Consultation requests, 28
Continuous quality improvement, 75, 77-81
Cost benefits, 85-90
Critical interventions, 21
Critical pathway, 98
- case management and, 91-94
- congestive heart failure, systolic dysfunction, 30-32
- coordinator, 99
- data collection log, 64
- definitions, 24
- development, 100

development team members, 99-100
- element analysis, 70-71

elements of, 50, 65-70
goal of, 2, 3
guidelines/procedures, 23-26
implementation, 100
management, 17-22
plan, 19-20
stages, 20-22
orientation to, 43-44
pneumonia, 89-90
policy statement exercise, 45-46
procedures, 25-26
process policy, 98-103
reference guides, 29-32
revisions, 77-81
steering committee, 98
systolic dysfunction heart
failure, 36-38
utilization, 100-101
Customer service, 7

Data accessibility, 12
Data analysis, 59-71
Data collection, 13, 47-58
log, 64
plan for, 57
process, 58
timing of, 57-58
Data identification, 49-50
Data management, 21-22
Day of care, 24
Decentralization, 9-10
Delinearizing process, 8-9
Discharge planning, 2, 3
Documentation, 26-28, 101-2
creation of, 28-29
pathway forms, 32-39
standardization of, 18

E-mail, 8-9
Episode of care, 57
Episode of care case management, 93
Exercise, policy statements, 45-46
Expert systems, 12

Feedback, 74-75
Financial benefits, 88
Financial costs, 88
Financial statements, 83-85
FOCUS, 78

Guideline implementation, 23-26

Health coordination case management, 93-94

Impediment removal, 75
Implementation cost impact, 88
Income statement, 84, 85
Individual plan of care, 27
Inductive thinking, 11
Information, types of, 26
Information specialist, 49
Information technology, reengineering and, 11-13
Institutional triggers, 76-77

Just-in-time education, 44-45

Kardex, 29

Leader, qualities of, 5-6

Medical care variance, 23
Medical executive committee, 99
Medical record information, 26
Mission statement, 76
Monitoring system, 47
Multidisciplinary team
education record, 38

plan of care, 28

Nursing education department, 99

One-time benefits and costs, 88
Organizational goals, 86
Outcome analysis, 70-71
Outcome measurements, 21, 68-69

Pareto chart, 68
Path/Builder/CaseMaster\TM, 22
Patient care review, 2, 4-5
Patient education
assessment, 38-39
materials, 18, 39-40
records, 28
Patient outcomes, 57, 63
Patient pathway, total hip replacement, 40-42
Patient variance, 24, 51, 98
PDCA, 79, 80
Performance reinforcement, 73-75
Physician orders
pre-printed, 28, 32-33
systolic dysfunction heart
failure, 35-36
Pilot test, 16
Pneumonia
community-acquired bacterial, 62
critical pathway cost benefit analysis, 89-90
Point of service, 24
Policy statements exercise, 45-46
Practitioner, 24
peer comparison, 67
triggers, 76
variance, 24, 51-52, 98
President, 98
Primary care case management, 93
Procedure implementation, 23-26
Process
reengineering, 4
triage of, 10-11
Profit and loss statement, 84
Progress notes, 29, 32, 34

Quality, cost benefit of, 85-90
Quality improvement, 2, 3

Random sampling, 22
Recording systems, 26-28
Reengineering, 1-2
case for action, 12-13
information technology in, 11-13
management's support of, 5-6
principles of, 3-11
process, 14-15
vision statement, 14
Reference guides, 29-32
Referral forms, 28
Reinforcement, 73-74
Revisions, 103
Revision team, 80
Risk management, 2, 3
Run charts, 65

Self-care case management, 92
Signals, 6
Skills building education, 44
Social service case management, 93
Software, 22
Staff education, 18
just in time, 44-45
orientation, 43-44
provision, 42-43
skills building, 44
Standing orders, 33
Symbols, actions taken, 6
System variance, 24, 51, 98

Systolic dysfunction heart failure
    critical pathway, 26-28
    multidisciplinary education record, 38
    physician orders, 35;36

Task
    assignments, 18
    combinations, 6-8
Total hip replacement
    outcome measurements, 69
    pathway intervention variance, 66
    patient pathway, 40-42
Total knee replacement, day D/C initiated, 66
Total quality management, 2
Triage, 10-11
Trigger identification, 76-77

Utilization review, 2, 3
Variance, 23-24, 66, 98
    decision model for, 52
    identification system, 52-53
    reasons for, 50-52, 67-68
    tracking system, 53-56
Vice presidents, 99
Vision statement, 14, 76

Work performance, 9-10